Pancreatitis Cookbook

Charles Thompson

Copyright© 2020by Charles Thompson

The information herein is offered for informational purposes solely, and is universal as so. The presentation of the information is without contract or any type of guarantee assurance. The trademarks that are used are without any consent, and the publication of the trademark is without permission or backing by the trademark owner. All trademarks and brands within this book are for clarifying purposes only and are the owned by the owners themselves, not affiliated with this document.

Contents

Pancreatitis Cookbook

Introduction

Pancreatitis is an inflammatory disease that affects the pancreas. It can occur in an acute or chronic form, and each year, about 500,000 patients in America alone are affected by this problem. This type of inflammation can be very dangerous by affecting a gland that performs a very important health task. In the acute form, pains are suddenly felt in the upper part of the abdomen, which can be accompanied, in very severe conditions, by nausea, vomiting, and fever. The pain can last for a few days, and it can affect the abdomen and reach behind the back. It can increase considerably after meals with a belly that is swollen and very painful. Pancreatitis is more frequent in men than in women; in the former, they are mainly caused by alcohol abuse - which in the Western world is the first cause of chronic pancreatitis ever - while in women, the most frequent cause is the presence of gallstones. Pancreatitis can be treated with pain relievers and an adequate diet to ensure good nutritional status. In the presence of complications, antibiotics are also used and, as a last resort, surgery.

Chapter 1: What is pancreatitis?

Pancreatitis is an inflammation of the pancreas, a large gland - located on the left, in the upper abdomen, behind the stomach and intestines - essential in maintaining the glycemic and digestive balance of the entire body. Pancreatitis can be acute or chronic. Both forms are severe conditions and can have serious complications. At first, pancreatitis manifests itself in an acute form and, if not treated, it can become a permanent disease (chronic pancreatitis). It is a serious condition that can cause dangerous complications and even death if it is not treated.

Acute pancreatitis, a form that occurs suddenly and usually resolves within a few days if properly recognized and treated at the hospital level (through intravenous hydration, antibiotics, and medicines to relieve pain). It is often linked to the presence of gallstones, and the most common symptoms are the presence of acute pain in the upper abdomen, nausea, and vomiting. To learn more about chronic pancreatitis, click here.

Chronic pancreatitis, a form that neither heals nor tends to improve; on the contrary, it worsens over time until it causes permanent damage. The most common cause is alcohol abuse, but it can also be caused by cystic fibrosis and other hereditary disorders, excessive concentrations of calcium and fat in the blood, some medicines, and autoimmune diseases.

Causes acute pancreatitis

The most common cause of acute pancreatitis is gallstones, small pebble-like formations made of solidified bile, which inflame the pancreas by passing through the common bile duct.

Another cause is the chronic consumption of alcohol in large quantities. Acute pancreatitis can occur within hours or up to two days of alcohol consumption.

Other causes of acute pancreatitis include:

- abdominal trauma,
- drugs,
- infections,
- tumors
- and genetic abnormalities of the pancreas.

Causes chronic pancreatitis

The most common cause of chronic pancreatitis is long-term alcohol abuse, but it can also result from an acute attack that damages the pancreatic duct. The damaged vent causes inflammation of the pancreas, from which scar tissue originates, and the progressive destruction of the gland.

Other possible causes of chronic pancreatitis:

- hereditary problems of the pancreas,
- cystic fibrosis, the most common inherited disease causing chronic pancreatitis,
- hypercalcemia (high levels of calcium in the blood),
- hyperlipidaemia or hypertriglyceridaemia (high levels of fat in the blood),
- some medications,
- some autoimmune conditions.

However, a large percentage of cases of chronic pancreatitis are idiopathic, that is, with no apparent cause.

Hereditary forms of pancreatitis can arise in individuals under 30 but may remain undiagnosed for several years. Intermittent episodes of abdominal pain and diarrhea lasting several days can progress to chronic pancreatitis. If the patient has two or more relatives in multiple generations with pancreatitis, it may be hereditary pancreatitis.

Risk factors

Men are more likely than women to develop inflammation of the pancreas.

Other risk factors include:

- familiarity with pancreatitis
- presence of gallstones
- diabetes
- obesity
- smoke

Symptoms

Acute pancreatitis generally begins with the appearance of a gradual or sudden pain in the upper abdomen, which sometimes also radiates to the back. The pain may be mild at first and worsen soon after meals. In most cases, it is intense, tends to become constant, and lasts for several days. The abdomen can be swollen and very painful. A person with acute pancreatitis typically appears and feels very ill and needs immediate medical attention.

Other symptoms include:

- swollen and painful abdomen,
- nausea and vomit,
- temperature,
- accelerated pulse.

Severe acute pancreatitis can cause dehydration and a drop in blood pressure. Eventually cardiac, pulmonary or renal failure may arise. Bleeding from the pancreas can lead to shock and even death.

Complications

Gallstones at the origin of acute pancreatitis must be surgically removed, together with the gallbladder.

In non-severe pancreatitis, cholecystectomy (removal of the gallbladder) can be performed during hospitalization.

In severe cases, the stones can be removed using ERCP. By directly visualizing the pancreas, gallbladder, and bile ducts, the stones can also intervene in acute and chronic pancreatitis complications. The cholecystectomy will then be performed later, a month or more after full recovery.

In case of infection, it may be necessary to drain the infected area, in fact, an abscess, through ERCP or surgery. Surgery may also be done for exploratory purposes to locate sources of bleeding, rule out pancreatitis-like conditions, or remove severely damaged pancreatic tissue. ERCP or endoscopic ultrasound also allows the drainage of pseudocysts formations of fluid and tissue residues that may form in the pancreas. If left untreated, enzymes and toxins in pseudocysts can enter the bloodstream and damage the heart, lungs, kidneys, or other organs.

Acute pancreatitis sometimes causes kidney failure. This condition requires periodic filtering (dialysis) of the blood or a kidney transplant. In rare cases, acute pancreatitis can cause breathing problems. Hypoxia can arise, a condition in which cells and tissues do not get enough oxygen. Hypoxia is treated with the administration of oxygen. However, some patients suffer from respiratory failure, despite oxygen administration and therefore require assisted ventilation for a certain period.

Chapter 2: Diet

The diet for acute pancreatitis varies considerably based on the severity of the disease.

In the most severe forms, it is better to avoid any form of oral feeding, both based on food and based on parenteral solutions (nasogastric tube).

This is necessary to keep the organ at rest which, in most cases, is unable to perform its endocrine function or its exocrine function adequately.

Nutrition for severe acute pancreatitis mainly occurs intravenously and is often associated with drugs of the type: analgesic, antibiotic, hormonal (insulin), etc.

The requirements of parenteral nutrition for severe acute pancreatitis are:

- High water content
- Concentration of carbohydrates proportional to glycaemia
- Low lipid content, mainly composed of medium-chain fatty acids
- Medium portion of essential amino acids
- Salts and vitamins in normal quantities.

In the milder forms, however, when the resolution is estimated in approximately 24 or 48 hours, it is possible to forego the intravenous nutritional administration by limiting the water compensation; in some cases, it is possible to start the food-based diet early.

For both situations, when the pancreatic enzyme levels are within the ordinary, it is possible to start with a solid diet.

The basic requirements of this diet are:

- TOTAL elimination of alcohol (including wine with meals) and drinks with other nerves (coffee, tea, energy, etc.)
- High splitting of total energy, with at least 6 small meals
- High water content
- High carbohydrate content, especially with a low glycemic-insulin index
- Low concentration of carbohydrates with a high glycemic-insulin index (especially in the case of diabetes mellitus)
- Low lipid content
- Modest protein content of animal origin, to be progressively increased.

Pancreatitis: What to eat?

When you suffer from pancreatitis it becomes necessary to review your weekly shopping and make substantial changes to your diet. To reduce the workload of the pancreas, it is therefore necessary to favor:

- Carbohydrates (potatoes, pasta, rice, toast), cereals and whole foods;
- Proteins understood as lean fish and white meats, such as chicken, turkey, veal, rabbit;
- Legumes, as long as you keep them in water, soaking them, at least from the previous evening and pass them through a vegetable mill once cooked, to make them more digestible;
- Vegetables, especially when cooked, blueberries and red grapes for the presence of resveratrol and antioxidants that help eliminate free radicals and reduce the symptoms of pancreatitis;
- Seasonal fruit, to fill up on vitamins, preferably ripe and, if possible, cooked, away from meals to facilitate digestion;
- Yogurt as a natural source of probiotics.

Pancreatitis: What not to eat?

In the presence of pancreatitis, there are a whole series of foods that should be avoided from the fridge, pantry and more, such as:

- All alcohol, spirits, caffeine and nicotine, absolutely counterproductive for pancreatic well-being;
- Aged cheeses, fatty or spicy, which tire the pancreas;
- Salami and sausages, with the exception of lean cooked or raw ham and bresaola (to be eaten in moderation anyway);
- Eggs and the preparations that contain them, such as mayonnaise and sweets;
- The cream, the bechamel and all the elaborate sauces;
- Molluscs, crustaceans, canned ;
- Particularly spicy foods;
- The fries.

It is also advisable to steam or grill food, or in the oven or a bain-marie; drink a lot of water during the day (the subject with pancreatitis often suffers from dehydration), also with the help of broths, soups, centrifuged, to satisfy the water need in the best possible way. Use sugar in moderation and prefer honey as a sweetener, where possible; finally, reduce extra virgin olive oil. To a teaspoon a day for seasoning food.

Chapter 3: Recipes for Breakfast

1) Crêpes of chickpea flour with cabbage and fermented cashew nuts

Ingredients:

For the crêpes:

- **280 g of chickpea flour**
- **500 ml of warm water**
- **40 g of extra virgin olive oil**
- **4 g cumin seeds**
- **4 g sage**
- **8 g of whole salt**
- **10 cabbage leaves.**

For the cashew spread:

- **150 g raw cashews**
- **20 g white miso**
- **8 g lemon juice**
- **10 g nutritional yeast**
- **3 g of whole salt**
- **3 g yellow mustard powder**
- **water q.s.**

For the crêpes: with the help of a whisk, mix the chickpea flour, water, and 20 g of extra virgin olive oil. Leave to rest for at least 8 hours. Then pick up the dough and season it with a mix obtained by blending the cumin, sage, and salt. Mix well. Heat a non-stick or iron pot well, pour a teaspoon of sunflower oil, and distribute it well over the entire surface. Pour a ladle of batter, cook it until it comes off, then turn it over and cook it on the other side as well.

When it is ready, place it on absorbent food paper and
proceed with the dough. Cut the cabbage leaves thin.
Heat a wok-like pan with the remaining extra virgin olive
oil. Sauté the cabbage for a few minutes, add salt and let
the vegetation water evaporate and it will come out.
Keep them aside. For the spread: soak the cashews for 12
hours at room temperature, changing the water at least a
couple of times. After that, rinse them well and put them
in a blender along with all the ingredients. Blend until the
mixture is creamy and without lumps. Serve the crêpes
with the cabbage, a few flakes of cashew spread, and
grated black pepper.

2) Stuffed chickpea flour pancakes

Ingredients:
- 3 heaping tablespoons of spelled flour
- 2 heaping tablespoons of corn starch
- 3 heaping tablespoons of chickpea flour
- 2 tablespoons of oil and 1 pinch of salt
- 1 pinch of nutmeg
- 300 ml of partially skimmed milk

For the stuffing
- 1 small thistle (about 200 g) already cleaned
- 1 slice of clean pumpkin
- ½ small leek
- 2 teaspoons of flour
- 2 teaspoons of lemon juice
- 4 tablespoons of oil and 1 pinch of salt

For the batter: dissolve the flour and starch in a little milk, then gradually pour the remaining liquid and oil, beating with a whisk. When the cream is thick and fluid, add the salt and nutmeg. Let it sit for 20-30 minutes.

For the filling: blanch the thistle in 500 ml of water where you have diluted the lemon and flour. Wash the leek and slice it thinly. Sauté it in a pan with 1 tablespoon of oil and 3 of water for 4-5 minutes, then add the coarsely grated pumpkin and the shredded thistle. After another 4-5 minutes turn off the heat. Mix the batter. Just grease a non-stick pan and pour a ladle of the mixture into a thin layer. Cook the crepes for a few minutes on both sides. Stuff them and close them in a bundle. Serve hot.

3) **Savory pie with red lentils**

Ingredients:
For the base (pan diameter 24 cm)
- **250 g wholemeal flour**
- **3 tablespoons of extra virgin olive oil**
- **a teaspoon of natural yeast**
- **a teaspoon of whole sea salt**
- **water q.s.**

For the filling
- **3 medium potatoes**
- **2 glasses of red lentils**
- **a clove of garlic**
- **a slice of ginger**
- **half a small pepper**
- **2 sage leaves**
- **extra virgin olive oil as needed**
- **whole sea salt to taste**
- **water or vegetable broth to taste**

To garnish the surface of the cake
- **Sesame seeds**
- **poppy seeds**
- **chopped almonds to taste**

In a large bowl, pour the flour, salt, and yeast and mix well. Make a hole in the center in which to put the oil and, a little at a time, the water needed to knead. Work vigorously until you have obtained a compact but soft, elastic, and not stiff dough. Let it rest for 30 minutes in the fridge. In a saucepan, boil some water with a handful of coarse salt and the unpeeled potatoes.

Cook them until they are soft. Drain them, let them cool and peel them. With a puree or a fork, mash them well. Mix well and set aside.

In the meantime, put a drizzle of oil in a saucepan, heat and fry the whole clove of crushed garlic and the chili pepper, add a little water, then add the finely chopped ginger, the sage, and the lentils previously washed under running water. Mix well and add the hot water or vegetable broth necessary to cover the lentils. Salt. Set aside more hot water or broth, which will be added during cooking. Usually, in 15-20 minutes, they are cooked, do not worry if they fall apart slightly. The flavor given to the cake does not vary. After cooking, let them cool. Roll out your base with the help of a rolling pin until you get an elastic dough, not too thin because it must support and give body to the cake. Line a baking sheet with parchment paper and lay the base on top, cutting off the excess edge, which you can use to prepare decorative strips for the surface. After removing the garlic and sage leaves, add the lentils to the potatoes. Mix well, seasoning with salt. Place the filling on the base, pour over a cascade of sesame seeds, chopped almonds, and poppy seeds. If you want, lay the puff pastry strips on top of the cake, forming the characteristic grid. Add a drizzle of oil on the surface and bake at 200 ° for about 40 minutes. Let it cool down a bit before serving. This savory pie is excellent when accompanied by raw and cooked seasonal vegetables.

4)   Energy cookies with oats and raisins

Ingredients:
- **300 g of rolled oats**
- **100 g of raisins**
- **the grated zest of a lemon**
- **the zest of a grated orange**
- **150 g of rice malt**
- **a teaspoon of ground cinnamon**
- **a teaspoon of vanilla powder**
- **apple juice to taste**

First, soak the raisins in warm water for about 15 minutes, turn on the oven at 180 ° and prepare a pan lined with parchment paper to lay the biscuits to cook them. Once this is done, you can dedicate yourself to the dough, starting with toasting the oat flakes in a hot pan for a few minutes, stirring often. Place them still hot in a large bowl in which you will add the grated citrus peel, cinnamon, vanilla powder, and finally, the well squeezed raisins. At this point, add the malt to the mixture; knead with your hands with the help of a little apple juice (just enough to be able to work the dough without making it too liquid). You can proceed by taking some of the dough to form balls that you will crush in your hands to give it the classic shape of a round biscuit. During this step, you can help yourself by wetting your hands with water. Place each biscuit in the pan and bake for about 10-15 minutes. Remove the pan from the oven and let the cookies cool. When they are cold, you can store them in an airtight jar, where they will keep well for a whole week.

5) Oat porridge with chocolate, cashew and orange

Ingredients:
- **about 10 tablespoons of oat flakes**
- **a few pinches of ground cinnamon**
- **a few pinches of vanilla powder**
- **2 tablespoons of rice syrup**
- **6-7 cashews**
- **dark chocolate to taste**
- **almond milk**
- **a slice of orange**

Put the oat flakes in a bowl, then pour enough milk to cover them abundantly. Let it rest in the fridge overnight. The next morning add the cinnamon, vanilla, rice syrup and mix well. Add more milk if necessary. Complete with crumbled or chopped cashews, dark chocolate into small pieces, and a slice of orange. Consume the porridge immediately.

6)   Pear, chocolate and hazelnut muffins

Ingredients:
- **3 cups of kamut**
- **2 tablespoons of cream of tartar**
- **half a teaspoon of ground cinnamon**
- **half a cup of toasted hazelnuts**
- **half a cup of dark chocolate**
- **half a cup of sunflower oil**
- **half a cup of wheat malt**
- **1 and a half cups of soy milk**
- **1 large cup of pears in small pieces**
- **1 pinch of salt**

Mix the flour, salt, cream of tartar, and cinnamon in a bowl; in another, emulsify the oil with the malt and milk, then pour it into the first, mixing everything without stirring much. Add the coarsely chopped hazelnuts and chocolate, the peeled and chopped pears. Spread the mixture into muffin cups and bake at 180 degrees for about 30 minutes.

Note: In this recipe, one cup is approximately 120 grams.

7)   Donut with carob flour

Ingredients:
- **340 g of water**
- **90 g extra virgin olive oil**
- **320 g wholemeal flour**
- **70 g carob flour**
- **50 g of corn starch**
- **1 sachet of gluten-free yeast**
- **9 dates and 9 plums**
- **90 g 92% dark chocolate**
- **1 pinch of salt**

Sift the flour, carob flour, yeast, corn starch, and salt.
Separately, blend the dates and plums with 140 g of
water. Emulsify this mixture with the rest of the water
and the oil. Combine the dry ingredients and create a soft
dough. Cut the dark chocolate with a knife and add to the
dough. Bake for about 40 minutes at 180 degrees.

8)   Chestnut flour muffins

Ingredients:
- **500 g of chestnut flour**
- **3 apples**
- **Apple juice**
- **½ teaspoon of cinnamon**
- **1 pinch of salt**
- **sunflower oil**
- **½ teaspoon of cream of tartar**

In a bowl, mix the chestnut flour, salt, cream of tartar, and cinnamon. Gradually pour in the apple juice necessary for a soft batter. Add the washed and sliced apples. Stir one last time. Brush a muffin pan with a little oil. Distribute the mixture and bake at 180 degrees for about 25 minutes. Remove from the oven and let them cool before serving.

9)   Radicchio and carrot muffins

Ingredients:
- **250 g of wholemeal flour**
- **1 carrot**
- **½ head of radicchio**
- **½ sachet of cream of tartar**
- **150 g of oat milk**
- **4 tablespoons of oil**
- **1-2 tablespoons of toasted linseed and sesame**
- **50 g of roasted peanuts**
- **1 pinch of salt**

Clean the radicchio, wash it and dry it, then cut it into thin slices. Wash the carrot and dry it, remove the ends and grate it. Gather the vegetables, seeds, and peanuts in a bowl. Separately, mix the flour with salt and yeast. Then add it to the bowl's contents, mix and gradually pour the milk and oil until you have a soft and creamy mixture. If it is too dry, add a little more oat milk. Pour the mixture into the appropriate cups and bake at 180 ° C for about 20 minutes. Serve the muffins warm or cold.

10) Apple and hazelnut tartlets

Ingredients:
- **200 g of hazelnuts**
- **200 g of almond flour**
- **100 g of powdered sugar**
- **250 g of peeled apples**
- **350 ml of water**
- **oil**

Finely chop the hazelnuts with the help of a food processor. Put them in a bowl and mix them with the lupine flour, icing sugar, and water. At this point, add the apples cut into small pieces and knead again, distributing the fruits evenly. Lightly oil the cake tins and arrange the mixture, leveling it well. Bake the cakes at 170-180 ° for about 35 minutes.

11) Smoothie with banana and tea

Ingredients:
- **1 banana**
- **almond milk**
- **1 teaspoon of tea**
- **a few pinches of vanilla powder**
- **rice syrup**

Peel the banana and cut it into small pieces. Put it in the glass of a hand blender or a mixer and mix until you get a puree. Add the tea, vanilla, and rice syrup and start the appliance again, adding enough almond milk to obtain a smooth and soft mixture. Drink it immediately.

12) Quinoa pancakes

Ingredients:
- **80 g of quinoa**
- **50 g of chickpea flour**
- **100 ml of water**
- **1 onion**
- **20 g of grated cheese**
- **salt**
- **extra virgin olive oil**

Rinse the quinoa and boil it for about 15 minutes in double its volume of water. Turn off, put the lid on and leave it to rest for another 10 minutes. It will be cooked when the grains, from white, become a little transparent. Let it cool down. Clean the onion and cut it into slices. In a bowl, prepare a batter with water, chickpea flour, Parmesan cheese, and salt. Add the cooked quinoa to the batter. You will get a fairly solid dough. Heat a little oil in a pan and pour a spoonful of batter. In contact with the heat, the batter will spread to form pancakes. A soup spoon of batter equals a pancake. You can cook 4 or 5 at a time, depending on the size of the pan. Let the pancakes set for a couple of minutes, then turn them on the other side. Serve hot.

13) Salty muffin

Ingredients:
- **130 g of wholemeal flour**
- **120 g of corn flour**
- **3 teaspoon of curry**
- **1 small carrot**
- **1 piece of leek (the green part)**
- **soya milk**
- **3 tablespoons of oil**
- **1 teaspoon of oregano**
- **3 tablespoon of mixed pumpkin, flax and sunflower seeds**
- **1 sachet of yeast**
- **salt**

Chop the seeds and put them in a bowl. Combine the two flours, curry, oregano, yeast, and salt. Pour in the oil first, then gradually add enough milk to have a soft mixture (about 1 glass). Complete with the diced carrot and the washed and thinly sliced leek. Pour the mixture into a tall, narrow mold lined with baking paper. Bake at 180 degrees for 35-40 minutes. When cooked, allow the muffin to cool, turn it out of the mold and let it cool. Serve with a thick tomato sauce or with chopped and sautéed leeks and carrots.

14) Kamut flour biscuits

Ingredients:
- **250 g of kamut flour**
- **150 g of maple syrup**
- **50 g of chopped and toasted almonds**
- **70 ml of corn oil**
- **50 g of raisins**
- **50 g of unsweetened cocoa powder**
- **20 g of yeast**
- **200 ml of warm water**
- **1 teaspoon of vanilla**
- **the grated peel of ½ orange**
- **1 pinch of salt**

In a bowl, combine the oil and maple syrup, mixing well. Gather the dry ingredients in a bowl: the flour, the chopped almonds, the unsweetened cocoa, the baking powder, the salt, and the vanilla, mix them evenly and add the raisins, water, and the mixture with the syrup. 'Maple. Work with your hands until you get a soft and smooth dough: lifting a bit of the dough with one hand and letting it fall slowly. Pour some of the dough into the pastry bag and squeeze to form corrugated discs on the pan (space the cookies apart, so they have room to rise). Bake the cookies in the oven at 200 ° for 20 minutes. Let them cool and serve them.

15) Cracker

Ingredients:
- **00 flour 500 g**
- **Extra virgin olive oil 120 g**
- **Dry yeast 4 g**
- **Salt up to 10 g**
- **Water 180 ml**

TO BRUSH
- **Extra virgin olive oil 3 tbsp**
- **Water 2 tbsp**
- **Salt up to taste**

Sift the flour into a bowl. Pour the water into a small bowl, add the yeast, and then stir for a few seconds until the yeast is completely dissolved. Pour the yeast and water mixture into the flour. The rest of the water dissolves the salt, then add the extra virgin olive oil to the flour and start kneading, adding the water a little from time to time. When you have blended all the ingredients, transfer the mixture onto a pastry board and knead until the mixture is smooth and homogeneous, to which you will give a round shape. Put the mixture obtained in a bowl and cover it with cling film. Let the dough rise for two hours until the initial volume is doubled. With the pasta machine, roll out the dough until sheets are no more than 2 mm thick. Cut the dough with a smooth pastry cutter to obtain 12 cm strips. Divide the stripes, and you will get the crackers to bake. With a skewer toothpick, make 5 holes in each of the crackers.

Line a dripping pan with parchment paper and place the shapes of the crackers on top, which you will lightly brush with an emulsion of water and oil; if you like, you can sprinkle the crackers with fine salt. Bake in a preheated static oven at 200 degrees for about 12 minutes (the crackers should slightly brown on the sides). As soon as you take them out of the oven, immediately remove them from the pan to prevent the latent heat from continuing to cook and darken them too much. Once cold, you can eat your crackers, sprinkle them with honey or jam!

Chapter 4: Snacks, appetizers and side dishes

1) Brussels sprouts with pears and walnuts

Ingredients
- **350 g of Brussels sprouts**
- **40 g of leek**
- **1 small pear**
- **60 g of shelled walnuts**
- **2 juniper berries**
- **salt**
- **4 tablespoons of oil**

Clean and wash the vegetables. Remove the most damaged leaves from the sprouts and divide them into four wedges; add them to the finely sliced leek, which you will dry for 5 minutes in a pan with 2 tablespoons of oil, half a glass of water, and the juniper. Cut the pear into cubes and coarsely chop the walnuts; add them to the mixture and continue cooking for another 3 minutes. Before removing from the heat, season with salt, season with the remaining oil, and stir.

2)   Slices of crispy bread with black cabbage and beans

Ingredients:
- **200 grams of dry beans**
- **300 grams of black cabbage**
- **10 slices of wholemeal bread**
- **7-8 cm of kombu seaweed**
- **a few sage leaves**
- **3 cloves of garlic**
- **extra virgin olive oil as needed**
- **Salt and Pepper To Taste**

Soak the beans overnight, remove the soaking water and cook them in plenty of cold water, with the kombu, sage and a clove of garlic, possibly in an earthenware pot, for about two hours or until tender. Low fire. Season with salt and pepper in the last 10 minutes of cooking; remove the kombu, sprinkle the beans with a drizzle of oil and set aside. Meanwhile, peel the black cabbage by removing the fibrous central rib, wash it well and cook the leaves immersed in lightly salted water, until tender (the black cabbage can be more or less tough). Drain, season with oil and a grind of pepper. Place the slices of bread in the oven and brown them on both sides. Rub them immediately with the remaining garlic. Place them on a serving dish and cover with the beans and black cabbage. Serve immediately.

3) Broccoli with miso sauce and nuts

Ingredients:
- **2-3 broccoli tops**
- **80 g of walnuts**
- **2 tablespoons of miso**
- **about 1 cm of ginger root**

Cut and wash the broccoli tops and place them in the steamer basket, adding a pinch of salt. Cook in a covered pot until the broccoli is tender but still bright green. Meanwhile, toast the walnuts in the oven at 180 ° until they are fragrant. Let them cool down. Chop them coarsely by hand to prevent them from releasing too much oil, and then grind them in a mixer with miso and water or vegetable broth, just enough to obtain a smooth cream. Flavor with the ginger juice, obtained by squeezing the grated root. Serve the vegetables with the sauce.

4)   Sweet and sour stewed pumpkin

Ingredients:
- **3 cups of chopped pumpkin**
- **2 tablespoons of extra virgin olive oil**
- **chopped sage to taste**
- **water q.s.**
- **2 tablespoons of rice vinegar**
- **salt**

Heat the oil in a pot with the chopped sage and rosemary, then add the pumpkin, a little salt and sauté for a few minutes. Add a little water and vinegar, cover, and let it simmer over low heat for about 15-20 minutes until the pumpkin is tender.

5) Quick pizzas

Ingredients:
For the dough
- **200 g of finely ground millet**
- **200 g of rice flour**
- **3 tablespoons of oil**
- **1 teaspoon of salt**
- **1 tablespoon yeast**
- **1 tablespoon of sesame and flax seeds**

For the filling:
- **500 g of clean pumpkin**
- **1 sprig of sage**
- **1 sprig of rosemary**
- **2 tablespoons of oil**

For the mini pizzas: Finely chop the seeds. Combine them with the other ingredients in a large bowl and knead with your hands to get a soft and homogeneous mixture. Let it rest for about 1 hour. For the filling. Cut the pumpkin into cubes, sprinkle with chopped sage and rosemary. Cook it in steam or the oven for 15-20 minutes, let it cool, and season with oil. Blend it until you have a cream, helping you if needed with a little water. Roll out the not too thin dough with a rolling pin and cut out discs with the help of a glass; place them on a baking sheet lined with parchment paper and cover with the cream. Bake at 170 degrees for about 15 minutes.

6)   Mushrooms with orange spinach

Ingredients:
- **400 g of fresh spinach leaves**
- **150 g of champignon mushrooms**
- **2 large handfuls of shelled almonds**
- **the juice of 1 blond orange**
- **oil**
- **white pepper, to taste**
- **pink Himalayan salt, to taste**

Clean the spinach and the mushrooms, which you will then have to slice thinly. Put the vegetables in a bowl with the peeled and chopped almonds and mix well. Season with orange juice, oil, a few pinches of Himalayan salt, and freshly ground pepper. Stir again and serve.

7) Quinoa with roasted carrots

Ingredients:

- **250 g of quinoa**
- **4-5 carrots**
- **4 shallots**
- **1/2 tablespoon of cumin**
- **1/2 tablespoon of turmeric**
- **1 handful of toasted pine nuts**
- **1 handful of parsley and very finely chopped celery**
- **extra virgin olive oil**
- **salt and pepper**

Peel the shallots and halve them; cut the carrots in four lengthwise and then into chunks. Put the vegetables in a pan seasoned with oil, cumin, and salt. Bake at 180 degrees for about 30 minutes, turning them now and then until they are well roasted. Meanwhile, wash the quinoa well in cold water, drain it in a tightly meshed colander and rinse again; drain well and dry briefly in a pan with two tablespoons of oil, turmeric, and pepper. Pour in boiling water equal to double the quinoa's volume, add salt, cover, and cook over very low heat for 15-20 minutes until the liquid is completely absorbed.

Shell the quinoa well and mix it with the vegetables, also collecting their cooking juices, with the pine nuts, celery, and parsley. Serve immediately.

8)   Spinach in a pan with dried fruit

Ingredients:
- **500 g of spinach**
- **50 g of dried apples**
- **50 g of raisins**
- **a little pine nuts**
- **1 clove of garlic**
- **extra virgin olive oil as needed**
- **Salt to taste**

Soak the apples and raisins for about 20 minutes in warm water. Clean and wash the spinach. Blanch them in lightly salted water for a few minutes. Drain them by squeezing them well, and cut them coarsely. Fry the garlic in a pan greased with oil, add the spinach, and after a while, the raisins and well-squeezed apples, pine nuts, and salt. Let it cook over high heat for a few minutes, season with salt, and serve the spinach hot.

9)   Crunchy and spicy chickpeas

Ingredients:
- **250 g cooked chickpeas**
- **5 g cumin powder**
- **5 g dry ginger powder**
- **8 g fine whole salt**
- **10 g rice flour**

Mix the spices, salt, and the powders . Put the chickpeas in a bowl and pour the mix. Using your hands, mix everything together so that the flour and spices stick to the chickpeas. Preheat the oven to 200 ° C. Place the chickpeas on a baking dish covered with baking paper. Bake for 20 minutes or until crisp.

10) Mashed fava beans

Ingredients:

- **250 g of broad beans**

- **1 white onion**

- **4 tablespoons of oil**

- **2 cloves of garlic**

- **salt**

Rinse the previously soaked broad beans overnight and boil them with the garlic for about 2 hours in a saucepan. Peel and chop the onion; put them in a large pan with a tablespoon of oil and a glass of water. Salt and cook over medium heat, uncovered, for about 10 minutes, until the liquid is used up. At the end, turn off and season with a little oil. Blend the beans and onion by immersion, season with the salt and the remaining oil; serve as a side dish.

11) Broccoli and tofu meatballs

Ingredients:
- **1 large or 2 small broccoli**
- **200 g of tofu**
- **1 tablespoon of barley miso**
- **1 tablespoon of oil**
- **breadcrumbs (if necessary)**
- **Sesame seeds**
- **salad of your choice**

Clean and wash the broccoli, including the stem (remove the hardest part). Steam it for a few minutes, just long enough to soften it, then chop it in a blender with the tofu, the miso dissolved in a little water from the vegetable and the oil; if the mixture is too soft, add some breadcrumbs a little at a time. Shape into balls 3-4 cm in diameter and pass them in the sesame seeds. Place them on a baking sheet lined with parchment paper and place them in a ventilated oven for 20 minutes at 180 °. Serve on a bed of shredded salad leaves.

12) Baked zucchini with curry

Ingredients:
- **5 zucchini**
- **4 tablespoons of pumpkin seeds**
- **1 tablespoon of chia seeds**
- **1 teaspoon of curry powder**
- **lemon juice**
- **black pepper**
- **extra virgin olive oil**
- **sea salt**

Wash the zucchini well and cut them into 4 lengthwise. Put them in a baking dish, sprinkle with oil, salt and bake at 180 °. Cook for about 25 minutes, turning them often. Let the vegetables cool slightly. Season with lemon juice, more oil if necessary, season with salt, pepper and complete with pumpkin and chia seeds, which you will distribute on the surface with the curry. Serve immediately.

13) Sauteed spinach with dried fruit

Ingredients:
- **500 g of spinach**
- **50 g of dried apples**
- **50 g of raisins**
- **a little pine nuts**
- **1 clove of garlic**
- **extra virgin olive oil as needed**
- **Salt to taste.**

Soak the apples and raisins for about 20 minutes in warm water. Clean and wash the spinach. Blanch them in lightly salted water for a few minutes. Drain them by squeezing them well, and cut them coarsely. Fry the garlic in a pan greased with oil, add the spinach, and after a while, the raisins and well-squeezed apples, pine nuts, and salt. Let it cook over high heat for a few minutes, season with salt, and serve the spinach hot.

14) Carrot puree with green olives

Ingredients:
- **500 g of carrots**
- **1 teaspoon of paprika**
- **2 teaspoons of cumin**
- **3 tablespoons of rice vinegar**
- **2 minced garlic cloves**
- **1 tablespoon of oil**
- **grated ginger juice**
- **green olives for garnish**
- **salt and pepper**

Peel and cut the carrots into rings and place them in a steamer basket. Cook them, covered, in a saucepan with lightly salted boiling water. After about ten minutes, check that they are soft. Blend them with the rest of the ingredients and a little cooking water to obtain a puree's consistency. Let the puree rest for a couple of hours so that the flavors blend. If you prefer, put it in the fridge for a while. Serve at room temperature or slightly chilled.

15) Croutons of bread with rosemary lentil cream

Ingredients:
- **Bay leaf 2 leaves**
- **Vegetable broth 400 ml**
- **Cloves 3**
- **Juniper berries 3**
- **Extra virgin olive oil 3 tbsp**
- **Salt up to taste**
- **Dried lentils 200 g**

FOR 10 CROUTONS
- **Vegetable Butter 80 g**
- **Baguette 10 slices**
- **1 sprig rosemary**

In a non-stick pan, fry the bay leaves, juniper berries, and cloves with a little oil over low heat. After 2 minutes, add the dried lentils. Cook everything for a few minutes, always over low heat; Wet the lentils with the broth, and continue cooking for at least 45/60 minutes, with the pot covered. Check often that the legumes do not dry out too much: in this case, add a few broth ladles. Once the lentils are ready, transfer them to a mixer, keep a little aside for the final garnish, reduce them to a cream, and then melt half of the butter provided in the recipe in a non-stick pan. Add the lentil cream, chopped rosemary, and a little water to the melted butter to make the cream itself more fluid; mix everything, being careful not to let the mixture dry out too much. Slice the bread and melt the remaining butter in another pan, in which you will toast the croutons for a couple of minutes, turning them on both sides.

Now transfer the lentil cream on each crouton, finally
garnish with a little of the lentils that you had kept aside,
with the help of a teaspoon and a few needles of
rosemary.

Chapter 5: Soups and salads

1)   Oat milk mushroom cream

Ingredients:
- **2 shallots**
- **2 tablespoons of flour**
- **400 ml of vegetable broth**
- **200 ml of oat milk**
- **400 g of mushrooms**
- **20 g of dried porcini mushrooms**
- **½ teaspoon of marjoram**
- **1 tablespoon of chopped parsley**
- **2 tablespoons of oil**
- **100 g of oat flakes**
- **salt**

Rinse the dried mushrooms and soak them in hot water for 30 minutes. Filter the liquid and squeeze the porcini mushrooms, then cut them up. Spread the flakes in a single layer on a baking sheet lined with baking paper, bake them at 180 ° and toast them for 10 minutes, turning them now and then. Let them cool. Meanwhile, you have cleaned the mushrooms with a damp cloth and sliced them. Chop the shallots and put them in a pan with a little broth, marjoram, and a pinch of salt. Let them soften over medium heat, then add the fresh and dried mushrooms. Stir, sprinkle with flour and pour in the hot oat milk without stopping stirring from avoiding lumps. Sprinkle with the rest of the hot broth and the soaking water of the porcini mushrooms. Cook the soup for about 20 minutes, then blend it by immersion. Season it with salt, season it with oil and transfer it to the soup plates, where you have distributed the toasted flakes. Garnish with parsley and serve.

2)   Spelled and potato soup

Ingredients:
- **250 g of spelled**
- **3 potatoes**
- **1 red onion**
- **1 heart of celery**
- **2 carrots**
- **100 g of peeled tomatoes**
- **extra virgin olive oil**
- **salt and pepper**

Soak the spelled in cold water overnight. The next day, rinse it and cook it in a pot with one and a half liters of salted water for about 20 minutes. Peel the potatoes and onion, peel the carrot and celery. Cut all the vegetables into cubes or small pieces. In an earthenware pot, first brown a fried onion, celery, and carrots with a salt pinch. Just wilted, add the potatoes and the broth until everything is covered . Stew on low heat. Halfway through cooking, pour in about a liter of broth and continue cooking for 20 minutes. Once cooked, pass the vegetables through a vegetable mill and add the boiled spelled. Mix the ingredients and season with salt and pepper. Serve the soup dressed with raw extra virgin olive oil.

3)   Carrot soup with almonds

Ingredients:
- **2 potatoes**
- **1 kg of carrots**
- **500 g of fennel**
- **1 stalk of celery**
- **150 g of almonds**
- **1 bunch of parsley**
- **2-3 tablespoons of sunflower oil**

Wash the fennel and celery, potatoes, and carrots; cut the prepared vegetables into small pieces and chop the almonds. Collect everything in a pot. Pour enough water to cover the vegetables by about two fingers. Bring to a boil, reduce the heat; cook for about 30 minutes, remove from heat, and work the mixture with the hand blender until creamy. Season with salt and complete with the washed and chopped parsley and sunflower oil.

4)   Pumpkin and cauliflower soup

Ingredients:
- **a small pumpkin**
- **half a teaspoon of salt**
- **a cup of cauliflower**
- **a teaspoon of white miso**

In a saucepan, arrange diced pumpkin. Cover with water, add salt and cook until the vegetables are well softened. Blend until you get a soft pumpkin cream. In a saucepan of boiling water, cook the pieces of cauliflower for 2-3 minutes. Drain and add them to the pumpkin cream. Dress with white miso. Garnish with parsley and serve.

5)   Spelled and bean soup

Ingredients:
- **120 g of beans**
- **150 g of pearl spelled**
- **1-2 tablespoons of extra virgin olive oil**
- **1 small leek**
- **2 celery sticks**
- **1 carrot**
- **1 piece of pumpkin**
- **1 potato**
- **about 2 liters of vegetable broth**
- **1 bunch of herbs (sage, rosemary, bay leaf)**
- **1 pinch of red pepper**
- **a small sprig of chopped parsley**
- **1 teaspoon of salt**

Soak the beans for 12 hours; remove the soaking water, cover abundantly with fresh water, bring to a boil; then cook for an hour and a half over low heat, adding salt towards the end of cooking. Take half of the beans with the cooking water and pass them through a vegetable mill. Cut the vegetables into cubes, toss the leek in the oil first for 1-2 minutes and then all the others with the salt and chilli. Add the spelled, the bunch of herbs and the vegetable broth; cook in a covered pot over low heat for 30 minutes. Add the beans (pureed and whole), and continue cooking for another 15 minutes. Let the soup rest for about an hour before serving (but it is also good right away!), Garnish each portion with a drizzle of oil and chopped parsley.

6) Colorful buckwheat salad

Ingredients:
- **300 g of buckwheat**
- **2 bay leaves**
- **250 g of boiled green beans**
- **4 ripe tomatoes**
- **1 large bunch of fresh basil**
- **100 g of green olives**
- **1 small clove of garlic**
- **200 g of canned corn**
- **oil**
- **salt and pepper**

Toast the buckwheat without adding fat and cook it with double the water for 20 minutes: when it boils, lower the heat and cook covered with salt and bay leaf. Drain it and let it cool. Meanwhile, wash the green beans, remove the seeds from the first and chop with the second. Rinse the basil well and blend it with the pitted olives, the chopped garlic in quarters, pepper, salt, and oil. Spread the dressing over the cereal, mix the other ingredients and serve this salad cold.

7) Coconut vegetable stew

Ingredients:

- **1 tablespoon of oil**

- **2 cloves of garlic**

- **1 fresh red pepper**

- **200 g of green beans**

- **250 g of cooked black beans**

- **2 potatoes**

- **400 ml of coconut milk**

- **the juice of 1 lime**

- **1 handful of fresh coriander**

- **2 handfuls of roasted cashews, lightly salted**

- **salt**

- **water**

- **cooked rice (optional)**

Heat the oil over high heat in a thick-bottomed saucepan. Brown the peeled the cleaned and chopped garli, red pepper, and potatoes, add salt and leave to flavor briefly, stirring constantly. Lower the heat, stir in the sprouted and chopped green beans, and if necessary, pour a little water, cover, and continue cooking for 5-10 minutes. When the potatoes are tender enough, add the black beans and coconut milk and cook. Once you have reached the consistency of a soft stew, remove from heat, sprinkle with lime juice, season with salt, mix and divide into plates. Complete with cashews and coriander washed and fragmented; serve with rice.

8)   Peach, parmesan and rocket salad

Ingredients:
- **2 yellow peaches**
- **80 g of rocket**
- **80 g parmesan**
- **7-8 tablespoons of extra virgin olive oil**
- **3 teaspoons of black sesame seeds**
- **salt**

Divide the peaches in half, remove the stone and peel them (if they are too ripe, peel them before halving and peeling them); then slice them thinly. Arrange the washed and dried rocket on four plates; distribute the prepared fruits and season the salad with oil and a light sprinkling of salt. Ultimate by distributing in each portion the pecorino reduced to flakes and sesame seeds.

9)   Cold avocado soup

Ingredients:
- **1 handful of fresh coriander**
- **1 clove of garlic**
- **a few tufts of chives**
- **the juice of 1 lime**
- **a few pinches of cumin powder**
- **a few pinches of nutmeg**
- **salt**
- **black pepper**

Combine the peeled and pitted avocados, the peeled and chopped garlic, the cleaned and chopped chives, the lime, the cumin, the nutmeg, salt, and pepper in a blender. Blend, adding cold water in small quantities until you reach a soft consistency. Add the washed and chopped coriander, work the mixture again to mix it, and transfer it to a bowl. Put it in the refrigerator to cool. Serve it in individual bowls, completing, if you like, with a little cream and a few leaves of fresh coriander or chopped chives.

10) Cream of spinach with pine nuts

Ingredients:
- **1 kg of spinach**
- **2 shallots**
- **500 ml of vegetable broth**
- **100 ml of soy milk**
- **100 g of creamy tofu**
- **2 tablespoons of flour**
- **2 tablespoons of pine nuts**
- **2 teaspoons of turmeric**
- **2 tablespoons of oil**
- **salt and pepper**

Clean the spinach, wash and drain them. Finely chop the shallots and let them soften in a saucepan with a little broth for about ten minutes. Add the flour, stir to avoid lumps, and add the spinach. Add salt, stir briefly and pour in the warmed milk and remaining broth, tofu, and turmeric. Cook for about ten minutes and blend by immersion. Peppered, seasoned with oil, and served garnished with lightly toasted pine nuts and, if desired, with oat cakes.

11) Radicchio and pear salad with ginger

Ingredients:
- **2 head of radicchio**
- **2 pears**
- **4 walnuts**
- **4 sprigs of parsley**
- **vinegar to taste**
- **1 piece of ginger**
- **3 tablespoons of oil**

Peel and wash the radicchio, then dry them with the centrifuge and cut them into strips not too thin. Gather them in a salad bowl. Add the chopped walnuts, the chopped parsley. Peel the pears and cut them into cubes. Mix them with the radicchio. Season with salt, vinegar, and oil. Peel and grate the ginger. Squeeze it very well in a cloth to extract all the juice, which you will pour on the vegetables. Stir and serve.

12) Cream of fennel and leeks

Ingredients:
- **300 g of clean fennel**
- **300 g of leeks**
- **½ teaspoon of chopped fennel seeds**
- **4 teaspoons of toasted sunflower seeds**
- **salt**

Wash the fennel and leeks well; of the latter, also use the green part. Finely slice the first courses, halve the second courses for a long time, and then cut them into slices or strips. Bring 800 ml of salted water to a boil and toss in the leeks. Blanch them for a minute, then add the fennel and fennel seeds, cover and cook gently for 15 minutes. Blend, put back on the heat, and simmer for a few minutes. Serve by distributing the sunflower seeds on the surface.

13) Barley and bean soup

Ingredients:
- **200 g of cooked beans**
- **150 g of pearl barley**
- **1 small onion**
- **1 small carrot**
- **1 stalk of celery**
- **100 g approx. of pumpkin pulp**
- **1 sprig of parsley**
- **1 clove of garlic**
- **4 tablespoons of oil**
- **1 pinch of chilli**
- **salt**

Boil the barley in 400 ml of water with a pinch of salt, for about 40 minutes, in a covered pot. Prepare a mixture of garlic, onion, celery, carrot, and parsley; cut the pumpkin into cubes. Fry the mixture in oil in a large pot with a pinch of salt; then add the pumpkin and let it simmer for five minutes, until softened, possibly with a little water. Then add the barley and beans with their cooking water or a little broth to get the right consistency (the soup should be creamy); bring to a boil and cook for another 5 minutes. Season with a pinch of chili and serve hot. Alternatively, you can cook the barley directly with the vegetables and add the beans towards cooking.

14) Chestnut and chickpea soup

Ingredients:
- **200 g of dried chestnuts**
- **200 g of chickpeas**
- **2 tablespoons of chopped parsley**
- **1 teaspoon of dried thyme**
- **1 clove of garlic**
- **2 shallots**
- **4 tablespoons of dry white wine**
- **1 teaspoon of fennel seeds**
- **1 bay leaf**
- **1 chilli**
- **3 tablespoons of oil**
- **salt**

Soak chickpeas and chestnuts separately for one night. Drain and rinse them. Put the first courses in a pressure cooker with the bay leaf and garlic. Cover them with water and cook for 15 minutes from the whistle. As soon as possible, carefully open the pot, add the chestnuts and then the fennel seeds and salt. Continue the pressure cooking for another 15 minutes. Meanwhile, peel and chop the shallots with the chilli. Sauté them in a pan with the thyme and wine. As soon as they begin to smell, turn them off and add them to the contents of the pot, which you will always have uncovered with caution. Continue cooking for another 10 minutes. Remove the bay leaf and blend almost all the chickpeas and chestnuts, using hot water if needed. Season with salt and season with oil. Serve the soup hot.

15) Spelled with avocado, orange and capers

Ingredients:
- **250 g of peeled spelled**
- **1 small avocado**
- **1 orange**
- **2 small handfuls of salted capers**
- **oil, to taste**
- **the juice of ½ lemon**
- **whole sea salt, to taste**
- **dried oregano, to taste**
- **white pepper, to taste**

Wash the spelled under cold running water and drain it. Cook it for about 45 minutes in filtered water, over low heat and with a lid, using 2 parts of water for one cereal part. Drain it and let it cool. In the meantime, clean the avocado, cut it into small pieces, peel the orange, divide it into raw peeled wedges, and then cut them into small pieces. Soak the capers in filtered water for 10-15 minutes, then rinse and squeeze them well. Add the already cooked spelled, cold or at room temperature, the avocado, the orange, and the capers in a salad bowl. Season with extra virgin olive oil, lemon juice, and salt, add the dried, chopped oregano and freshly ground pepper, and mix well. Serve immediately, or keep the spelled salad in the refrigerator until ready to serve.

Chapter 6: Single course

1)   Ricotta and walnut pie

Ingredients:
- **500 g of ricotta**
- **4-5 tablespoons of lightly toasted walnuts**
- **2 tablespoons of milk**
- **4 nice pinches of saffron stigmas**
- **3 tablespoons of marjoram leaves**
- **salt**
- **oil for the molds**

Infuse the saffron in hot milk for about an hour. Pour the infusion over the ricotta you have sifted into a bowl, add the coarsely chopped walnuts and marjoram, season with salt. Mix all the ingredients to form a cream that you will distribute in the individual round casseroles about 10-12 centimeters wide, greased with a drizzle of oil. Bake for 20 minutes at 180 degrees. When the patties are ready, take them out of the oven and gently remove them from the molds; arrange them in the center of the plates, accompanying them with salads arranged in a crown and possibly dressed with a light vinaigrette.

2)   White bean paté with caper pesto

Ingredients:
- **300 g cannellini beans (cooked weight)**
- **30 g of onion**
- **30 g of Evo oil**
- **20 g of salted capers**
- **15 g of lemon juice**
- **10 g of lemon zest**
- **a bay leaf**

Boil the beans, which you have previously soaked for at least 12 hours, with a bay leaf. Soak the capers in plenty of warm water and leave them to desalt for the entire preparation time. Then reduce them to a puree, mashing them with a fork or blending them with a hand blender. Help yourself with half the oil and lemon juice to make the pate more homogeneous and fluffy. Separately, chop the onion and cut the lemon zest into thin strips. Drain the capers and chop them coarsely. Place the pate on a plate, season it with the remaining extra virgin olive oil, onion, lemon peel, and capers. Serve at the table cold or room temperature, accompanied by slices of toasted bread.

3)   Chickpea stew

Ingredients:
- **a cup of chickpeas left to soak overnight**
- **2 teaspoons of extra virgin olive oil**
- **2 carrots**
- **2 cloves of garlic**
- **2 celery sticks**
- **2 bay leaves**
- **2-3 tablespoons of miso**

Drain the chickpeas and cook them in a pot full of water for about an hour over medium heat. Cut the vegetables and brown them in a pan with oil for about 5 minutes over high heat. Add the vegetables and bay leaves to the beans and simmer until the vegetables are well cooked. Add the miso and cook for a few more minutes. Serve with a sprinkling of chopped parsley.

4)   Pasta and cauliflower

Ingredients:
- **350 g of wholemeal short pasta**
- **1 cauliflower of 800 g**
- **400 g of peeled tomatoes**
- **3 tablespoons of oil**
- **2 cloves of garlic**
- **1 teaspoon of marjoram**
- **50 g of Parmesan cheese**

Clean the cauliflower, wash it, divide it into florets and steam it for 10-15 minutes. Meanwhile, put the crushed tomatoes with a fork, chopped garlic, marjoram, salt in a saucepan. Cook them for about 15 minutes. Add the cauliflower. Cook for a few minutes, stirring. Bring water to boil in a saucepan.

When it comes to the boil, cook the pasta for the time indicated on the package. Drain and pour the cauliflower pasta. Grate the cheese, turn the heat back on under the pasta and stir for 1 minute over medium heat. Season with oil, season with salt, and serve.

5) Eggplant stuffed with mushrooms

Ingredients:
- **4 medium eggplants**
- **300 g of champignon mushrooms**
- **1 clove of garlic**
- **1 small bunch of fresh thyme**
- **bread crumbs**
- **3 tablespoons of oil, salt**

Wash and clean the eggplants, dry them and divide them in half lengthwise. Dig them inside with a sharp knife, being careful not to break the shell. Cut the pulp into cubes and cook in a pan with a little water. Add salt, stir for a few minutes over medium heat. Cook for 10 minutes. Clean and slice the mushrooms. Stew them in a pan with the peeled and halved garlic and 1 tablespoon of oil. After 15 minutes on low heat, turn off and add salt. Mix the mushrooms with the eggplant pulp and season with the remaining oil. Season with salt and complete with chopped thyme. Fill the eggplants with this mixture and sprinkle them with breadcrumbs. Arrange them on a baking sheet lined with parchment paper and bake at 190 ° for 40-50 minutes. Serve warm or hot.

6) Pasta with cherry tomatoes and capers

Ingredients:
- **280 g of wholemeal pasta of your choice**
- **12-15 cherry tomatoes, cleaned and quartered**
- **4-5 tablespoons of extra virgin olive oil**
- **half a white onion, peeled and chopped**
- **1 generous handful of salted capers**
- **1 handful of fresh, clean oregano**

Soak the capers in cold water for about 20 minutes, rinse and drain. Cook the pasta in abundant salted water. Meanwhile, heat the oil in a large pan and lightly soften the onion. Add the tomatoes and cook the capers for 4-5 minutes beforehand. Once the pasta is cooked, drain and add it to the sauce. Stir a couple of minutes, remove from heat, stir and serve.

7)   Zucchini stuffed with chickpeas

Ingredients:
- **4 medium-large zucchini**
- **vegetable broth q.s.**
- **250 g of boiled chickpeas**
- **2 shallots**
- **1 teaspoon of coriander seeds**
- **20 g of dried mushrooms**
- **1 teaspoon of marjoram**
- **the juice of 1/2 lemon**
- **3 tablespoons of oil**
- **Salt to taste**

Soak the mushrooms in warm water for 30 minutes. Wash the zucchini and steam them whole for 5 minutes. Let them cool, tick them, and cut them in half lengthwise; gently dig them to remove most of the pulp, taking care not to break the peel. Set them aside. Finely chop the shallots and let them soften for a few minutes in a pan, lightly covered with broth. Add the marjoram and the squeezed and thinly sliced mushrooms. Follow with the crushed coriander and salt. Cook for 10 minutes on low heat, finally adds the chickpeas, a tablespoon of oil, and lemon juice. Stir and turn off the heat. Blend by immersion, helping you if needed with a little broth but trying to keep the mixture firm. Transfer it to the zucchini shells, which you will then line up on a baking sheet lined with baking paper. Bake at 180 degrees for about 30 minutes. Serve the dish hot or warm, seasoned with the remaining oil.

8)   Rice and peas

Ingredients:
- **200 g of rice**
- **1 Kg of peas**
- **garlic**
- **parsley**
- **extra virgin olive oil**
- **salt and pepper**

Bring salted water to a boil for cooking the rice.
Meanwhile, in a pan, cook the shelled peas cold with
finely chopped garlic and parsley and a glass of water.
When almost cooked, evaporate any excess water, add
salt, and season with extra virgin olive oil. Serve the
boiled rice with the peas.

9)   Pasta with chickpeas and celery pesto

Ingredients:
- **250 g of pasta**
- **150 g of cooked chickpeas**
- **70 g of tender ribs and celery leaves**
- **50 g of linseed or sesame seeds**
- **50 ml of water from pasta or legumes**
- **oil and salt**

Prepare the pesto. Lightly toast the flax (or sesame) seeds in a non-stick pan. After a couple of minutes, turn off the heat. Peel the celery and wash it, dry it and chop it. Put it in the hand blender's jar with the seeds and water from the pasta (or chickpeas). Add lightly salt and stir, gradually adding the oil needed to obtain a soft cream, similar to cream. In the meantime, you will have boiled the pasta al dente. Drain it, mix it with the chickpeas and season with the celery pesto, then serve it.

10) Spaghetti with walnut and basil sauce

Ingredients:
- **400 g of spaghetti**
- **100 g of shelled walnuts**
- **80 g of pine nuts**
- **1 clove of garlic**
- **30 g of basil leaves**
- **2 tablespoons of grated parmesan**
- **3 tablespoons of oil**
- **salt**

Prepare the sauce. Spread the walnuts and half of the pine nuts on a baking tray in a single layer. Bake them at 150 ° for about ten minutes until they are lightly toasted. During this time, stir them a couple of times. Let them cool down and remove the skin by rubbing them. Put them in a mixer with a little salt and chop finely. Add the peeled and chopped garlic, then washed and dried basil, a few tablespoons of hot water. Continue to work the ingredients until they are homogeneous, adding a little more hot water. Complete with oil. Cook the spaghetti in boiling salted water, and season immediately with the walnut and basil sauce. Sprinkle them with the grated Parmesan and serve.

11) Artichoke and lentil cake pan

Ingredients:
- **12 artichokes**
- **1 lemon**
- **300 g of lentils**
- **2 shallots**
- **1 sprig of rosemary**
- **1 sprig of sage**
- **1 teaspoon of thyme**
- **vegetable broth**
- **bread crumbs**
- **4 tablespoons of oil**
- **salt**

Soak the lentils overnight, rinse them and place them in a saucepan with the chopped rosemary and sage. Cover them with cold water and cook for about 40 minutes. Add salt only at the end. Clean the artichokes, halve them and wash them in water acidulated with lemon juice. Cook them al dente in a pan with the thyme, a tablespoon of oil, and a little water, salt. Be careful not to break them and keep them crunchy. Blend the lentils until the mixture is not too moist. Finely chop the shallots, let them dry in a pan with a tablespoon of oil and a little water. Add the past and let it flavor for a few minutes. Add another tablespoon of oil and stir. Grease a round mold with high sides, and sprinkle it with breadcrumbs. Form the first layer with half of the artichokes. Pour half of the remaining oil, distribute the legume purée and arrange the rest of the artichokes on the surface. Season with the remaining oil and bake at 190 ° for 10 minutes. Serve the dish hot.

12) Brown rice with ginger

Ingredients:
- **400 g of cooked brown rice**
- **2 spring onions**
- **1 carrot**
- **cabbage 350 g**
- **2 tablespoons of oil**
- **salt**
- **1 piece of ginger root**

Cut the spring onions into rings, the carrot into not too thin matches, and the cabbage into strips. Grease a pan with oil and toss the spring onions with a pinch of salt for a minute. Then add the carrot, cabbage, and another pinch of salt and sauté for another 8-9 minutes, often stirring, until the vegetables begin to be tender (possibly add a couple of tablespoons of water). Then add the cooked rice and a little water to the pan's bottom, cook covered for 5 minutes. Finally, season with the ginger juice, mix, and serve.

13) Baskets of potatoes with zucchini and cheese

Ingredients:
- **Potatoes 300 g**
- **Zucchini 200 g**
- **Mozzarella g**
- **Extra virgin olive oil as needed**
- **Salt up to taste**
- **Oregano to taste**

Peel the potatoes and then cut them into 1 mm thin slices. Transfer them to a bowl and season with olive oil, salt, and oregano. Stir to flavor well and then butter 12 aluminum molds; arrange the potato slices first on the bottom and then on the inner edges to completely cover the molds. Now place them on an oven rack and cook in a preheated convection oven at 200 ° for 20 minutes. Meanwhile, cut the mozzarella into cubes, wash and trim the zucchini, then cut them into cubes. In a pan, pour the oil and add the zucchini, add salt and cook for 15 minutes over medium heat. After cooking, keep aside. Meanwhile the baskets will have finished cooking, take them out of the oven. Stuff the baskets with a few cubes of mozzarella, then with the zucchini, and finish with a last layer of mozzarella. At this point, put it back in the oven for 10 minutes, just long enough to melt the mozzarella. Turn out the potato baskets, let them cool slightly, and then serve them on the table.

14) Potato pie in a pan

Ingredients:

- **Potatoes (about 1) 180 g**
- **Parmesan to grate 40 g**
- **Zucchini flowers 6**
- **Mozzarella 100 g**
- **Raw ham 100 g**

First, wash and dry the potatoes in their skins, slice them thinly and store them in a bowl full of water to prevent them from turning black. Take the zucchini flowers and cut off the stem, and detach the leaves from the flower base. To remove any earth residues inside the flower, gently wipe with a brush. Open the flower and remove the pistil. Cut the mozzarella into cubes and set aside. Now drain the potato slices and dry them with a cloth, heat a non-stick pan and arrange the first layer of potatoes on the spiral bottom, lay the potatoes overlapping them once you have made a circle, place a potato in the center so that there are no empty spaces between the slices. Sprinkle the whole surface with some of the cheese. Cover with the lid and heat for about 2-3 minutes. Spread another layer of potatoes in a spiral as you did previously, continue with a layer of cheese to cover the entire surface. Now stuff with half of the sliced ham, half of the zucchini flowers, and even half a dose of mozzarella cubes. Continue with the remaining raw ham and the remaining zucchini flowers covered with the remaining mozzarella cubes and more cheese. Cover with the lid and let everything cook for about 10 minutes. Serve the potato pie in the pan immediately, so you can still enjoy it racy!

15) Saffron risotto

Ingredients:
- **Saffron in pistils 1 tsp**
- **Rice 320 g**
- **Vegetable butter 125 g**
- **Parmesan cheese to be grated 80 g**
- **Water q.s.**
- **Vegetable broth 1 l**
- **Salt up to taste**

First, put the saffron pistils in a small glass, pour enough water over the pistils to completely cover the pistils, mix and leave to infuse overnight; in this way, the pistils will release all their color. Then prepare the vegetable broth; for the recipe, you will need a liter. In a large pan, pour 50g of butter taken from the total dose required, melt it over low heat, then pour the rice and toast it for 3-4 minutes, so the grains will seal and keep cooking well. Next, proceed with cooking for about 18-20 minutes, adding the broth a ladle at a time, as needed, as the rice absorbs it: the grains must always be covered. Five minutes before the end of cooking, pour the water with the saffron pistils that you had infused, stir. Once cooked, turn off the heat, add salt, stir in the grated cheese and the remaining 75 g of butter, mix and cover with the lid on, let it rest for a couple of minutes. At this point, the saffron risotto is ready; serve it hot.

Chapter 7: Fish

1) Crispy salmon

Ingredients:
- **Salmon fillet (4 of 250 g each) 1 kg**
- **Bread 100 g**
- **1 sprig parsley**
- **Dill 1 sprig**
- **Thyme 4 sprigs**
- **Rosemary 2 sprigs**
- **Lemon zest 1**
- **Extra virgin olive oil 50 g**
- **White pepper in grains 1 tsp**
- **Salt up to taste**

First, prepare the breading: cut the bread into pieces and put it in a mixer, then add the dill, the peeled thyme, the needles of rosemary and parsley. Pour in the oil too, then add the lemon zest, salt and white pepper. Blend until you get a coarse consistency. Now take care of the salmon fillets: remove the skin with a thin-bladed knife and remove the bones with the help of a kitchen tongs, then transfer the fillets to a drip pan lined with parchment paper and cover them with the breading, making it adhere well with your hands. . After covering the fillets evenly, cook in a preheated convection oven at 190 ° for about 20 minutes. After the cooking time, take out and serve your crispy salmon hot!

2) Baked salmon

Ingredients:
- Salmon steaks (4 pieces) 660 g
- Potatoes 170 g
- Lemon zest 1
- Lemon juice 25 g
- Dry white wine 25 g
- Extra virgin olive oil 50 g
- Parsley to chop 1 tbsp
- Salt up to taste
- Black pepper to taste

To prepare the baked salmon, first remove the fish bones with tweezers and check that there are no bones left by sliding a fingertip on the pulp. Remove the spine with a knife, then roll one end on itself and wrap the other end around the slice to obtain a medallion. Tie the medallion with a kitchen string to ensure that it maintains the shape even during cooking and transfer the medallions on a baking sheet lined with parchment paper. Take a fairly regular shaped potato, wash it and cut it into thin slices with a mandolin, without peeling it: the slices must be no more than 1 mm thick otherwise they will not be cooked enough. Now take care of the emulsion: grate the zest of a lemon in a bowl, then add 25 g of lemon juice, oil, white wine, chopped parsley, salt and pepper and mix well with a fork. Season the salmon medallions with part of the emulsion, then cover them with the slightly overlapping potato discs and sprinkle the potatoes with the remaining emulsion.

When the medallions are ready, bake in a preheated static oven at 180 ° for about 20 minutes, then operate the grill at 240 ° and continue cooking for another 3-4 minutes, until the potatoes are golden. After the cooking time has elapsed, remove the cooking string and immediately serve your delicious baked salmon!

3)   Mediterranean-style salmon fillets

Ingredients:
•**Salmon 800 g**
•**Dried oregano 1 sprig**
•**Extra virgin olive oil 30 g**
•**Salt up to taste**
•**1 clove garlic**
•**Pitted black olives 70 g**
•**Pickled capers 5 g**

In a large bowl, add the peeled and halved garlic and the chopped dried oregano. Add the oil, salt, and mix. Take the salmon steak, remove the bones with tweezers, remove the skin if present; then cut into 4 fillets of equal thickness. Arrange the salmon fillets on a baking dish, and with a teaspoon, arrange the garlic oil. Season with salt, add the black olives and capers. Bake in a preheated static oven at 180 ° for about 15 minutes (if you want to use the convection oven, bake at 160 ° for about 10 minutes). After this time, take out and serve your still warm Mediterranean salmon fillets!

4)   Tuna tartare

Ingredients:
•Tuna in slices 450 g
•Oranges 1
•Extra virgin olive oil 40 g
•Salt up to taste
•Black pepper to taste
•Shortcrust pastry 230 g
•Wild fennel 3 sprigs

Start grating the zest of an orange, then cut it in half and squeeze the juice. In a bowl, pour the extra virgin olive oil, the orange juice and its zest. Finely chop the fennel, keeping a few strands aside for the final decoration, add it to the mixture and emulsify with a whisk. Meanwhile, prepare the shortcrust pastry shells. Adjust the emulsion with a pinch of pepper and salt. Prepare the shortcrust pastry shells that will be used to make tartare single portions: roll out the shortcrust pastry (you can use a roll of already made shortcrust pastry), cut out 10 circles of about 10 cm in diameter and line 10 round molds with a diameter of 8 cm , after having buttered them. Prick the bottom with the tines of a fork and cook in white, covered with dried legumes as weight, in the oven at 180 degrees for 10-15 minutes. When they are golden, take them out of the oven, let them cool and turn them out. Take the tuna steaks: make sure you have bought especially fish. It is recommended to freeze it for 96 hours at -18 degrees and then defrost it for use in the recipe. Rinse and dry the tuna fillets with absorbent paper. Cut them into small cubes half a centimeter thick and place them in a large bowl.

Pour the oil and orange emulsion over them and mix so
that the tuna is well flavored. Then fill the cakes with one
or two tablespoons of tuna tartare and decorate your
tartare with a few sprigs of fennel.

5)   Tuna in pistachio crust

Ingredients:
- **Tuna 600 g**
- **Poppy seeds 1 tbsp**
- **Extra virgin olive oil 3 tbsp**
- **Breadcrumbs 20 g**
- **Chopped pistachios 50**
- **Dried tomatoes in oil 30 g**
- **Salt up to taste**

Get yourself a slice of fresh tuna, place the slice in the freezer for at least an hour so that it is more convenient to cut without breaking the fibers. Remove the tuna from the freezer and cut it lengthwise into slices about 2-3 cm thick. Put the tuna slices in a baking dish and drizzle them with the olive oil. Meanwhile, dry the dried tomatoes with a cloth to remove excess oil and chop finely with a knife. Place the chopped pistachios in a bowl, add the chopped tomatoes, poppy seeds and breadcrumbs. Stir to mix the ingredients well and salt the breading to taste. Take the slices of tuna and pass them in the breadcrumbs, pressing well on all sides. Place a couple of tablespoons of extra virgin olive oil in a non-stick pan and once the necessary heat is reached, add the breaded tuna slices and cook them for 1 minute per side, turning them only once. Do not continue cooking so that the tuna remains pink inside, the tuna must not turn white otherwise the meat will be harder. Remove the pistachio crusted tuna from the pan and cut into 2 cm thick slices, then place them on a serving dish and serve immediately.

6)   Baked sardines

Ingredients:
- **18 sardines for a total of about 250 g**
- **Breadcrumbs 60 g**
- **Extra virgin olive oil 60 g**
- **1 sprig parsley**
- **Thyme 1 sprig**
- **1 clove garlic**
- **Grated Parmesan cheese 20 g**
- **Pine nuts 30 g**
- **Extra virgin olive oil to grease the pan 15g**

Pour the breadcrumbs, grated cheese and the crushed garlic clove into a bowl. Rinse, dry and finely chop the parsley; then also add it to the breading and further flavor with the thyme leaves; pour the 60 g of oil and mix everything until you get a uniform mixture. At this point take a baking dish measuring 19x15 cm and sprinkle it with about 15 g of oil. Arrange the sardines horizontally without overlapping each other, salt (not excessively), pepper and cover with half of the previously prepared mixture. Arrange another layer of sardines, taking care to position them vertically (opposite to before), salt, pepper and cover the entire surface with the remaining part of the breading. Finish by decorating the surface with pine nuts. Then cook the sardines in the oven in grill mode at 200 ° for 8 minutes, until they are golden brown. Once cooked, serve the baked sardines while still hot.

7)   Orange mackerel

Ingredients:
•Mackerel (4 whole clean) 1200 g
•Orange peel 1
•Extra virgin olive oil q.s.
FOR MARINATING
•Orange juice
•Extra virgin olive oil 30 g
•Dill 2 sprigs
•2 cloves garlic
•Black peppercorns 1 tbsp
•Salt up to 1 tbsp

Make diagonal cuts on the sides of the mackerel and set aside. Take care of the ingredients for the marinade: with the back of the spoon, crush the peppercorns so they will release their aroma better, then squeeze the juice from the oranges. Peel and thinly slice the garlic. Grease a baking dish with oil, place the mackerel on top and season them on the surface with another drizzle of oil, the peppercorns, salt, scented with the sprigs of dill and flavored with the slices of garlic. Finally, sprinkle the fish with half of the orange juice, cover with plastic wrap and leave to marinate for 2 hours in the refrigerator. After the marinating time, go to cooking: heat a pan with a drizzle of olive oil and, when it is hot, lay the fillets. Let them cook over high heat for 4 minutes without touching them, then turn them, sprinkle them with the remaining orange juice and continue cooking for another 2 minutes. Once the sauce has congealed and the mackerel are well flavored, serve them immediately garnishing them with grated orange zest on the surface.

8)   Mackerel in foil

Ingredients:
- **Mackerel (2 clean mackerel)**
- **Celery 90 g**
- **Yellow peppers 70 g**
- **Eggplant 50 g**
- **Lemons 1**
- **Basil to taste**
- **Extra virgin olive oil q.s.**
- **Salt up to taste**

Chop the celery and cut it into cubes, then cut the eggplants into slices and cut into cubes. Remove the internal seeds and the stalk of the pepper and cut it first into strips and then into cubes. Transfer all the cut vegetables to a bowl, scented with fresh basil leaves and season with oil, salt. Now place each clean mackerel on a 35x31 cm sheet of parchment paper, fill the belly of the mackerel with a spoonful of vegetables and then distribute the rest around the fish. Season the fish with a drizzle of olive oil. Wash the lemon and cut into thin slices, then place 3 lemon slices on top of each mackerel. Now close the parcel by lifting the flaps of parchment paper and placing them on top of the fish, then seal well by folding the sides. Place the packets on a baking tray lined with parchment paper and bake in a preheated static oven at 200 ° for 20 minutes. When cooked, take your mackerel in foil out of the oven and serve hot.

9)   Swordfish carpaccio with green and pink pepper

Ingredients:
- **Swordfish 500**
- **Semi-skimmed milk 250 g**
- **Pink peppercorns 5**
- **Green peppercorns 10**
- **Extra virgin olive oil 50 g**
- **Himalayan salt (pink) 5 g**

Start by cutting the swordfish slices. Cut the swordfish steak into 16 slices of about 30 g each and 3-4 mm thick. To facilitate the operation, keep the swordfish steak to compact it in the freezer for an hour before slicing it. If you don't have a slicer available, buy the swordfish already cut into slices for the carpaccio or have it cut in your trusted fish shop. Remove the skin of the swordfish with a knife and arrange the slices in a baking dish. Start preparing the marinade: pour the milk and oil into a bowl. Add the green peppercorns, pink pepper and pink Himalayan salt. Emulsify the mixture with a whisk to mix all the ingredients. Pour the marinade into the pan where you have placed the swordfish slices and cover with plastic wrap. The carpaccio must marinate in the refrigerator for at least 4 hours. After this time, remove the swordfish carpaccio from the fridge and, with the help of a spatula, lift the slices of swordfish one by one, draining the marinade a little, and place them in an ovenproof dish. Bake at 180 degrees for no more than 5 minutes, so that the the fish releases the absorbed marinade. Stir in the swordfish carpaccio with green and pink pepper before serving.

10) Cod fillet with ginger

Ingredients:
- Cod fillet 400 g
- Salt up to taste
- Black pepper to taste
- Extra virgin olive oil 50 g
- Lime zest 1
- Lime juice 10 g
- Fresh ginger (pulp) 20 g
- Mint a few leaves

FOR THE RICE
- Basmati rice 200 g
- Coconut milk 400 g
- Water 200 g
- Coarse salt 1 tbsp
- Cinnamon sticks 1
- Curry 1 tsp

Grate the lime zest in a bowl and squeeze it into juice and pour 10 g into the same bowl. Peel the ginger and grate it, then collect the pulp with a spoon and place it in the bowl with the lime, pour in the olive oil and stir to mix the sauce. Take the cod fillets and place them on a baking sheet lined with parchment paper, salt them and spread the sauce on the surface. Bake in a preheated static oven at 220 ° for 25 minutes. Meanwhile, prepare the rice: pour the basmati rice into a pan, add the coconut milk, the coarse salt, the curry and a stick of cinnamon. Pour in the water, cover with the lid and bring to a boil, then lower the heat and cook for 15 minutes until the liquids are completely absorbed. When the rice has absorbed the liquids, turn off the heat and remove the cinnamon stick.

Meanwhile, the cod will be cooked, take it out of the oven and serve it accompanied with the spiced basmati rice, garnishing with mint leaves.

11) Salad rolls stuffed with tuna

Ingredients:
- **Tuna fillet 100 g**
- **Lettuce 4 leaves**
- **Broad beans 400 g**
- **Extra virgin olive oil 40 g**
- **Basil 3 leaves**
- **Salt up to taste**
- **Low-fat yogurt 20 g**
- **Chopped pistachios to taste**
- **Chives 8 strands**

Shell the beans and collect them in the mixer's glass, pour the olive oil, and blend to obtain a cream. Also, add the yogurt, salt, and mix with a spoon to combine. Scent, the cream with the chopped basil, leaves with your hands. In a pan with a drizzle of oil, brown the tuna for a few minutes. Now take the lettuce leaves, wash them well under running water, then dry them thoroughly with a cloth. Divide each leaf in half, taking care to remove the more rigid central core. Take one half of the lettuce leaf, spread the cream of beans and yogurt, and the entire leaf and stuff with the cooked tuna cut into chunks. Roll up the leaf, tie it with a thread of chives to seal the roll. Garnish with chopped pistachios to taste and continue in the same way for all the others. Your salad rolls stuffed with tuna are ready to be brought to the table. Accompany them with an extra cream of broad beans!

12) Cod with yogurt and purple potatoes

Ingredients;
- **Cod 400 g**
- **Natural white yogurt 120 g**
- **Purple potatoes 200 g**
- **Extra virgin olive oil 60 g**
- **Salt up to taste**
- **Thyme to taste**
- **4 slices bread**
- **Vegetable butter 40 g**

Take the cod fillets, and boil them in a pot for about 10 minutes, until they are white and tender. Pour the potatoes into cold water and cook for about 15 minutes from boiling. Then drain and peel them. In a blender, pour the cod and purple potatoes, peeled and coarsely cut into pieces, add the extra virgin olive oil, season with salt and start blending everything. Keep running the mixer while adding the white yogurt, then work until you get a smooth and whipped cream. Add the thyme leaves. Transfer the mixture to the fridge for at least 10-15 minutes. Cut 4 slices of bread, then take the butter and spread it on the bread, then arrange them on a dripping pan lined with baking paper and toast the slices in a static oven preheated to 200 ° for about 10 minutes, until they are golden brown. Serve your creamy cod mousse with yogurt and purple potatoes on the toasted bread, and add a few thyme leaves.

13) Tuna with sesame

Ingredients:
- **Tuna (4 fillets) 150 g**
- **Black sesame seeds 10 g**
- **White sesame seeds 20 g**
- **Extra virgin olive oil 35 g**
- **Lemon juice 25 g**
- **Salt up to taste**

In a dish, pour the sesame seeds, and mix them. Take the tuna: we recommend that you make sure that the tuna you have purchased has been slaughtered; however, we recommend that you freeze it for at least 96 hours at -18 degrees, then defrost it before using the recipe. Pass the slices of tuna over the seeds to bread them on both sides as evenly as possible. Heat a non-stick pan and only when it is hot, place the breaded tuna fillets and cook over high heat for 1 minute, then turn them with a spatula, continue cooking for another minute. Once seared, the tuna will be raw inside, but you can extend the cooking according to your taste if you like. Once cooked, transfer the fillets to a cutting board, immediately cut them into slices, and serve immediately.

14) Sea bream with carrots and zucchini

Ingredients:
- **Sea bream 2 pieces (clean)**
- **Extra virgin olive oil 30 g**
- **Carrots 150 g**
- **Zucchini 150 g**
- **Thyme to taste**

Wash and peel the carrots, then trim the ends and cut them into slices of about 5 mm thick. Wash and trim the zucchini, too, cut them in half lengthwise and then further divide each half; finally, cut them into cubes of about 1 cm thick. Pour the oil into a large non-stick pan and when it is hot, place the sea bream inside, then add the carrots, the zucchini, the spring onion, and the sprigs of thyme, and add salt. Cover the pan with a lid and cook over medium heat for 7 minutes, then turn the sea bream with the help of 2 spatulas, being careful not to break them; cover again with the lid and cook for another 7 minutes. Of course, cooking times may vary depending on the weight of the sea bream you will use. The pan-fried sea bream is ready to be served!

15) Swordfish and broccoli medallions

Ingredients:
- **Swordfish fillet 400 g**
- **Broccoli 200 g**
- **Potatoes 400 g**
- **Marjoram 3 sprigs**
- **Extra virgin olive oil q.s.**
- **Salt up to taste**

Put two pans with water to bring to the boil; in one place, the thoroughly washed potatoes when the water is still cold, when it boils, calculate for about 30-40 minutes. Meanwhile, wash the broccoli, put them in the other pan when the water has boiled, and simmer for about 5 minutes. Then drain the broccoli and chop coarsely with a knife, then let them cool. When the potatoes are cooked, peel and mash them with a potato masher in a large bowl, then preheat the oven to 200 ° in static mode. Finally, take the swordfish fillets, cut them into cubes, and then chop them coarsely with a knife. When the vegetables have cooled, take the bowl where you mashed the potatoes, add the chopped broccoli and swordfish, salt, and add the marjoram leaves, then mix with your hands to mix all the ingredients. Take some dough and shape it with a 6.5 cm diameter pastry ring to form the medallions: with these doses, you should get 6. Transfer the medallions on a baking tray lined with parchment paper, season with a drizzle of oil, then bake them in a preheated static oven at 200 ° for about 20 minutes.

Chapter 8: Meat

1) Salad baskets with turkey

Ingredients:
- **Turkey breast 250 g**
- **Baby lettuce 100 g**
- **Cashews 25 g**
- **Carrots 1**
- **Parsley to taste**
- **Extra virgin olive oil q.s.**

Place the turkey breast on a cutting board and cut it into irregular pieces. Then take a non-stick pan, heat a drizzle of oil. Add the turkey breast bites and salt. Cook the morsels for about 10 minutes, turning them from time to time to cook them inside until they are golden brown. When the turkey morsels are cooked, transfer them to a mixer, operate for a few seconds until the meat is well chopped, and then transfer the blended mixture into a large bowl. At this point, place the cashews on a cutting board and chop them coarsely. Sauté the chopped cashews in a non-stick pan and toast them for a few minutes, until crisp and darker. Then add the toasted cashews to the chopped turkey bites. Then take a carrot, peel it and divide it in half. After that, slice it into tiny cubes. Also, wash the parsley under running water and chop finely on a cutting board. At this point, add the diced carrot and chopped parsley to the mixture. Now wash the salad carefully and leaf it through, placing the crispest and most curved leaves on a serving dish. Then proceed to fill them with the dough. Your baskets of lettuce with turkey are ready to be served.

2) Meatballs in sesame crust

Ingredients:
- **Minced veal 300 g**
- **Wholemeal bread crumb 65 g**
- **Parmesan (for grating) 50 g**
- **Sesame seeds 50 g**
- **Black sesame seeds 25 g**
- **Eggs 1**
- **Salt up to taste**

Cut the wholemeal bread crumb into cubes, removing the outer crust, and crumble it in a mixer. In a large bowl, pour the veal, mixing them with your hands; add the chopped breadcrumbs, then the grated cheese. Incorporate the egg and season with salt. Mix with your hands until you get a homogeneous mixture. Each and continue like this until you finish the mix available: with our doses, you will have to obtain 38 meatballs. Pour the white sesame seeds into a tray and add them to the black sesame seeds, mixing them carefully. Pass the meatballs over the sesame, making it stick well to the meat. Continue in this way with all the remaining meatballs and, once finished, arrange them side by side on a baking tray lined with baking paper. Bake the meatballs in a preheated static oven at 180 ° for about 25 minutes, seasoning them with a drizzle of oil if necessary. After the required time, take out of the oven and enjoy your sesame-crusted meatballs hot.

3) Veal slices with mushrooms

Ingredients:

- **Veal (walnut) 400 g**
- **Champignon mushrooms 500 g**
- **Vegetable butter 50 g**
- **00 flour 40 g**
- **Extra virgin olive oil 10 g**
- **Salt up to taste**
- **Thyme to taste**
- **1 sprig chopped rosemary**

Take the veal slices, and with the meat mallet, slice them to make them thinner, flour the veal slices on both sides, and then shake them to remove the excess flour. Now take care of cleaning the mushrooms: with a small knife, begin to remove the earthy part on the stem, scraping it gently until any traces of earth are removed. If the mushroom is clean enough, remove the few earth residues with a brush, do not wash them with water to not spoil them. Slice the mushrooms and set them aside. Now proceed with cooking the meat: In a pan, melt half a dose of butter (25 g), adding the olive oil; once melted, lay the floured veal slices, add salt and brown them for 3 minutes per side or until a crust forms. Once golden brown, let them cool on a plate and take care of the mushrooms: In the same pan in which you cooked the meat, melt the other half of the butter, season with the chopped rosemary, add the sliced mushrooms and sauté over medium heat for two minutes , then add salt. At this point, add the veal slices browned and kept aside and flavored with the thyme leaves, cook over low heat for a minute, adding a ladle of water if necessary, and serve the veal with the mushrooms very hot!

4)   Milk chicken breasts

Ingredients:
- **Sliced chicken breast 4**
- **Vegetable butter 40 g**
- **Extra virgin olive oil 10 g**
- **00 flour q.s.**
- **Skimmed milk 170 g**
- **Salt up to taste**
- **Thyme 4 sprigs**

Arrange the slices on a cutting board and, using a meat mallet, beat them to obtain thin slices. Arrange the oil and butter in a pan, let it melt gently, and in the meantime, flour the chicken slices. As you move them into the pan, raise the heat slightly and wait about 2 minutes until a nice crust has formed. Then turn the slices, wait a couple of minutes again, pour the milk first, and then the thyme leaves into the pan. Add salt, cover with a lid and let it cook for another 4-5 minutes until the milk has thickened. At this point, you just have to serve your milk-filled chicken breasts still hot!

5) Roasted rabbit

Ingredients:
- **Rabbit in pieces 1.2 kg**
- **Rosemary 4 sprigs**
- **Salt up to taste**
- **Vegetable broth 2000 g**
- **Potatoes 800 g**
- **Thyme 4 sprigs**
- **Bay leaf 1 leaf**
- **Extra virgin olive oil 80 g**

Chop the rosemary, then transfer half of it into a pan where you have poured 40 g of oil. Add a bay leaf and let it cook over low heat for 2-3 minutes. Raise the heat, and add the rabbit pieces; let them brown on both sides for 3-4 minutes. Add a ladle of broth and cook over low heat for another 5-6 minutes. In the meantime, prepare the potatoes: peel them and cut them into rather large chunks. Transfer everything to a bowl, flavor with the chopped rosemary needles, and set aside the thyme leaves and salt. Drizzle with 20 g of oil and mix. Transfer everything to a large pan, oiled with about 10 g of oil, so that the potatoes are well distributed. Then also arrange the previously browned rabbit pieces. Add the remaining vegetable broth and cook the rabbit with the potatoes in a preheated static oven at 200 ° for 40 minutes. Once out of the oven, serve your rabbit in the oven while still steaming!

6)   Turkey chunks with saffron

Ingredients:
- **Turkey breast 600 g**
- **Saffron (one sachet) 0.15 g**
- **Water about 140 g**
- **Extra virgin olive oil 10 g**
- **Potato starch 1 tsp**
- **00 flour q.s.**
- **Salt up to taste**

FOR THE ASPARAGUS
- **Asparagus 400 g**
- **Water 100 g**
- **Extra virgin olive oil 10 g**
- **Salt up to taste**

Start by cleaning the asparagus: wash them, dry them, remove the toughest end, cut them diagonally, and keep them aside. Heat the oil in a pan, add the asparagus, add salt and cook over medium heat for 7-8 minutes, adding about 100 g of water to keep the vegetables from drying out. Once they are cooked, keep them aside and take care of the turkey. Cut the turkey breast into strips and then cut them into cubes of about 1.5-2 cm. Heat a little oil in a pan. Meanwhile, flour the diced turkey in a sieve so as to remove the excess flour. Once the oil is hot, add the turkey, let it brown and then wet with about 100 g of water, or just enough to keep the turkey from drying out. Dissolve the saffron in a little warm water and add it to the preparation; add salt, stir and continue cooking; the morsels must cook in total for about 10 minutes; the time may vary according to their size.

Make a cream to thicken the preparation: pour a teaspoon of starch into a small bowl, dilute it with a couple of tablespoons of water and mix to obtain a homogeneous mixture. Add the melted starch to the still hot preparation and mix. Your chicken nuggets with saffron are ready; serve them accompanied with a side of asparagus.

7)   Chicken strips with radicchio

Ingredients:
- **Chicken breast 650 g**
- **400 g long radicchio**
- **Brown sugar 30 g**
- **Water 100 g**
- **Extra virgin olive oil 10 g**

FOR MARINATING
- **Extra virgin olive oil 50 g**
- **Thyme 2 sprigs**
- **Marjoram 2 sprigs**
- **Salt up to taste**

Take the chicken breast, cut it in half, and make some pretty thin strips. Pour the oil into a pan, add the thyme and marjoram leaves, and season with salt. Distribute the strips of chicken next to each other in the pan so that the marinade is evenly distributed; cover with cling film and refrigerate for at least 2 hours. Wash the radicchio with plenty of fresh running water; remove the base, cut it in half, remove the hard edge, and then cut it into strips lengthwise. In a pan, add the water, the brown sugar and cook for another 2 minutes. Also, add the radicchio cut into strips and cook for 2 minutes, raising the heat. Remove the chicken from the refrigerator and add it to the vegetables. Cook for 2-3 minutes and, when the chicken turns brown, turn off. Finally, you can serve and taste your chicken strips with radicchio.

8)   Loin of rabbit mashed carrots

Ingredients:
- **12 rabbit loins**
- **5 carrots**
- **Vegetable broth 2 spoon**
- **Oil**
- **Salt**
- **Vegetable butter 1 teaspoon**

Heat three tablespoons of oil, add the diced carrots and two tablespoons of broth, cook, and add salt. Remove and blend until you have a smooth cream. Heat four tablespoons of oil and a knob of butter, place the rabbit loins in it, brown them evenly, salt them at the end. Remove them and cut each loin into two or three pieces. On the bottom of the serving dish, pour the carrot purée and, on top, the rabbit loins. Serve.

9) Chunks of chicken in fennel sauce

Ingredients:
- **Chicken breasts g 600**
- **Fennel n 3 medium**
- **Garlic cloves 2**
- **Dry oregano 1/2 tsp**
- **Chopped onion 4 tbsp**
- **Extra virgin olive oil**
- **Salt and pepper**

In a large skillet, heat the oil and quickly brown the diced chicken over high heat. Brown on all sides, then drain and keep warm. In the same pan, add the chopped onion, garlic, and cook over low heat for a few minutes. Add the cleaned, washed, and thinly sliced fennel. Wet with two water glasses, add the salt, and oregano, cover, and simmer for about 20 minutes or until the water has dried, and the fennel is almost reduced to cream. Bring the chicken back on the heat, stir, and cook for another 5 minutes. Turn off and serve hot.

10) Roast turkey stuffed with broccoli

Ingredients:

- **Turkey breast 700 g**
- **Broccoli tops 250 g**
- **1 egg white**
- **Garlic 1 clove**
- **1 pinch chili**
- **2 tablespoons olive oil**
- **Salt to taste**

Preheat the oven to 180C. In a pot filled with salted water, boil the broccoli until tender. Drain just ready. In a pan heat 1 tablespoon of oil and brown the minced garlic for a few minutes. Add the tops of boiled broccoli and the chili pepper. Cook for a few minutes, until they are well flavored. Turn off and let cool, then add the egg white and mix well. On the cutting board, roll out the turkey breast, cut a side pocket, and stuff with broccoli. Close with kitchen string, brush with the rest of the oil and inform at 180 ° for 40 minutes. Turn once. If necessary, moisten with a little broth. Remove from the oven and leave to rest for a few minutes, then slice and serve hot.

11) Turkey burger

Ingredients:

- **Wholemeal hamburger buns 4**
- **Ground turkey 600 g**
- **Aubergines 480 g**
- **Auburn tomatoes 320 g**
- **Green salad 60 g**
- **Rosemary to taste**
- **Oregano to taste**
- **Thyme to taste**
- **Salt to taste**
- **Black pepper to taste**
- **Extra virgin olive oil 10 g**

Start by chopping the aromatic herbs: rosemary, oregano, and thyme. In a bowl, add the minced meat with the mince; season with salt and pepper. Knead all the ingredients by hand and let the mixture rest in the refrigerator for 15 minutes. Meanwhile, wash and tick the aubergine removing the ends. Slice it about half a centimeter thick and place it on a well-heated and lightly greased plate. After a few minutes of cooking, turn the aubergine discs so you will also cook them on the other side at the end of cooking, set aside. Browse your salad and rinse it thoroughly to get rid of soil residues, then transfer the lettuce onto a tray with paper towels and gently dab it to dry; in this way, you will not damage it. Finally, wash the tomato and slice it in half centimeter thick slices after having stripped it of the stalk. At this point, all your ingredients are ready.

Take the minced meat from the fridge and place it inside an 11 cm circular pasta bowl that you will have placed on a parchment paper sheet. Then help yourself with the back of a spoon to level the surface to smooth and brush each hamburger with a little oil.

Place the meat medallions on the hot grill, and after 4 minutes of cooking, you can turn them with the help of a spatula to cook them on the other side for the same time. If you want a well-warmed and slightly toasted sandwich, cut the bread into two parts, then arrange the two parts on the still hot grill, letting go for a few minutes, until the base has become crispy. As soon as your sandwiches are hot, switch to the composition: then on the sandwich base lay 3-4 lettuce leaves and 4 tomato disks, then 4 slices of aubergines and finally your meat medallion. Close with the other half of bread, and your turkey burgers are ready to be bitten still hot!

12) Chicken and green beans rolls

Ingredients:
- **Chicken breast (8 slices of 30g) 240g**
- **Fresh green beans 100 g**
- **Raw ham (8 slices) 70 g**
- **Salt up to taste**
- **Extra virgin olive oil 15 g**

FOR THE YOGURT POTATO SALAD
- **Potatoes 500 g**
- **White yogurt 100 g**
- **Partially skimmed milk 20 g**
- **Chives 3 strands**
- **Salt up to taste**
- **Black pepper to taste**

Pour the potatoes into a saucepan with plenty of cold water, place it on the stove and let it boil, then cook the potatoes for 20-30 minutes depending on their size, doing a test with a fork. The potatoes will be cooked as soon as they no longer resist, at which point drain them and let them cool a little, then peel them and let them cool. Once the boiled potatoes are completely cooled, cut them into pieces of a couple of centimeters. Collect the cubes in a container and pour the yogurt together with the chives that you can cut with scissors and mix. If you notice that the mixture becomes too thick, dissolve by adding 1-2 tablespoons of milk, season with salt and pepper, mix, and place in the refrigerator, covering with cling film.

Meanwhile, tick the green beans, then remove the two ends, rinse them under running water and blanch them in plenty of boiling water for 10-15 minutes. Then drain the green beans and let them cool a little, adding a little cold water to stop cooking, so they will remain a nice green color. Finally, arrange the green beans in a bowl and season with salt. Arrange the slices of chicken breast on a cutting board and salt them only on the surface. Just above the center, place a handful of green beans. Starting from the highest part, roll the chicken slice with the green beans in the middle to roll up the meat on itself and thus obtain a roll; repeat the operation for all the other slices. Insert two toothpicks for each roll; in this way, you will be sure that it does not open during cooking. Pour extra virgin olive oil into a pan and when it is hot, place the rolls, turning them over after a few minutes of cooking over high heat and continue to seal the meat well. Let them cool for a few moments, and do not throw away the cooking oil that will be used later. Remove the wooden skewers from each roll and salt the surface that was not previously salted. Arrange the slices of raw ham on a cutting board and starting from the bottom roll the slice all around the roll so that the ham completely covers the roll and does so for everyone. In a baking dish, pour the rolls' cooking juices and place them in them, letting them cook in a static oven preheated to 180 ° for 15 minutes. As soon as the chicken and green bean rolls are cooked, you can serve them with your yogurt potato salad!

13) Turkey steak with fennel and pomegranate

Ingredients:
- **Whole turkey breast 800 g**
- **Fennel 400 g**
- **Pomegranate (1 medium) 400 g**
- **Extra virgin olive oil 80 g**
- **Black pepper to taste**
- **Salt up to taste**
- **Dill to taste**
- **Salt to taste**

On a hot plate, pour a drizzle of oil. Place the turkey on it and cook over medium heat on the first side for about 25 minutes. After the first 25 minutes, turn it over and cook for another 25 on the other side. In the meantime, prepare the dressing: take the pomegranate, cut it in half and shell it, collecting the beans in a bowl; keep some aside for the final decoration, pour the others into a mixer, and blend. Then pass the puree obtained through a colander to filter the juice you can put in a tall glass. Add 40 g of oil, salt, and pepper. Blend everything. Wash and trim the fennel to remove the green part. Divide it in half, then slice it finely, then transfer it to a bowl to the season with 30 g of oil, salt, and pepper. Flavor with the chopped dill with your hands. Stir and spread on a serving dish. Take the turkey, cut it to a thickness of about 1 cm for each slice, and distribute it on the bed of fennel. Season with the pomegranate seeds kept aside sprinkle with the pomegranate and oil emulsion; your sliced turkey with fennel and pomegranate is ready to be served.

14) Baked chicken legs with apples

Ingredients:

- Chicken legs (4 spindles) 500 g
- White wine 50 g
- Extra virgin olive oil 40 g
- Salt up to 10 g
- Sweet paprika to taste
- Black pepper in grains to taste
- Pink peppercorns to taste
- White pepper in grains to taste
- Juniper berries to taste
- Parsley to taste
- Sage as needed
- Rosemary to taste
- Thyme to taste

FOR APPLES

- Fuji apples (about 2) 500 g
- Brown sugar 5 g
- Salt up to 5 g
- Water 50 g
- ½ lemon juice

Start by finely chopping the parsley, sage, rosemary, and thyme, and set aside. Put the black, white, and pink peppercorns and juniper berries in a mortar and press them with the pestle to reduce them to powder. Put the chopped herbs and ground spices in a jug, pour the olive oil, add 10 g of fine salt, the wine, and flavor with sweet paprika, then mix with a spoon to flavor.

Take an ovenproof dish and grease the bottom with olive oil, place your chicken thighs next to each other here, then cover them with the previously prepared minced spice. Cook the legs in a preheated static oven at 180 ° for 45 minutes. In the meantime, wash and dry the apples, cut them first in half and then into quarters, and finally cut them into smaller and irregular pieces. Pour the apple pieces into a pan, add the brown sugar, 5 g of fine salt, and sprinkle with half a lemon juice. Cook over medium heat to dissolve the sugar, then pour in the water, lower the heat and continue cooking for 10 minutes until the apples are soft. Meanwhile, even the chicken will have finished cooking and will be golden on the surface, so take out and immediately serve your chicken legs in the oven with apples!

15) Chicken with tomatoes and avocado

Ingredients:
- **Chicken breast 550 g**
- **Extra virgin olive oil as needed**
- **Salt up to 1**
- **Black pepper 1 tsp**
- **Lime 1**
- **Oregano 1 tsp**

FOR THE SIDE
- **Copper tomatoes 500 g**
- **Avocado 200 g**
- **Red onions 100 g**
- **Salt up to 1 tsp**
- **Paprika 1 tsp**
- **Black pepper 1 tsp**

First, cut the chicken breast into slices, beat them with a meat mallet to make them thinner. Transfer the meat to a pan, then season with oil, salt, and pepper. Also, add the lime zest and its juice, finally flavored with oregano. Mix well to flavor. Cover with cling film and set aside until ready for cooking. Now take care of the tomatoes: after having washed and dried them, cut them into wedges, and then cut them into cubes. Peel and chop the red onion. In a bowl, combine the tomatoes and onion. Now divide the avocado in half, cut the pulp vertically, and then horizontally to obtain cubes. Pour the avocado into the bowl. Season with oil, paprika, salt, and pepper. Now go to cooking: heat a grill well, place the chicken breasts, and cook for 5 minutes.

Then turn them and continue cooking for another 5 minutes. Once cooked, immediately serve the chicken with the diced tomatoes and avocado.

Chapter 9: Dessert

1) Buckwheat and dark chocolate cake

Ingredients:
- **100 g dates**
- **200 g buckwheat**
- **60 g bitter cocoa**
- **90 g 95% dark chocolate**
- **Grated orange peel to taste**
- **140 g tofu**
- **½ teaspoon of agar agar**

Soak the buckwheat for 24 hours, then drain and place in a sprouter. Rinse twice a day for 2-3 days, and as soon as it begins to sprout, place in the dryer basket at 42 ° for 8 hours. Blend the sprouted and dried buckwheat, dates, vanilla, and grated orange zest at maximum power. Add the tofu and continue blending. Separately, dissolve the agar agar in cold water and add to the mixture, mixing again. Add the dark chocolate in pieces and bring to a boil for a few minutes. Pour the mixture into a square shape, a level well, and store in the freezer for 3 hours. When the cake is ready, sprinkle with cocoa. Let it rest out of the freezer for at least half an hour.

2) Beetroot brownies

Ingredients:
- **2 boiled beets**
- **200 g semi-wholemeal flour**
- **100 g dark chocolate (80-90%)**
- **50 g extra virgin olive oil**
- **50 g rice malt**
- **16 g yeast**
- **flaked almonds to taste**
- **1 handful of toasted hazelnuts**

Grate the beets, melt the chocolate in a bain-marie, add the oil, the malt, add the beets and mix everything. Add the sifted flour and baking powder. Mix well until the mixture is quite thick and soft. At this point, add the toasted hazelnuts and coarsely cut them with a knife. Transfer the dough to a previously greased square baking dish (about 30-40 cm). Bake in a preheated oven at 180 ° for about 30 minutes.

3) Lactose-free strawberry ice cream

Ingredients:
- **500 g of clean organic strawberries**
- **the juice of 1/2 lemon**
- **100 g of rice syrup**
- **260 ml of unsweetened rice milk**

Cut the strawberries, sprinkle them with the lemon juice and rice syrup, mix and let them rest in the refrigerator for half an hour. After this time, blend the mixture briefly with the rice milk. Leave it to cool for another half hour. Operate the ice cream maker and pour the mixture. It will take between 20 and 25 minutes to get good ice cream, be divided into cups or glasses, and be enjoyed immediately.

4) Coconut balls

Ingredients:
- **1 cup of cashews**
- **5 dates**
- **grated coconut to taste**
- **rice milk to taste**

Pitted the dates, cut them into small pieces, put them in a robot together with the cashews, and blended them finely. With your hands, form balls, compacting them well. Let them rest for half an hour in the fridge. Meanwhile, mix a little coconut with two tablespoons of rice milk. Take the balls back and roll them in this mixture until they are evenly covered. Finally, put them in the paper cups and serve them.

5) Pear and cinnamon cake

Ingredients:
- **140 g of type 0 wheat flour**
- **160 g of millet flour**
- **1 p of sea salt**
- **½ teaspoon of yeast**
- **4 medium pears (2 quite ripe, 2 firmer)**
- **about 160 ml of rice milk**
- **100 ml of oil**
- **180 g of rice malt**
- **½ teaspoon of ground cinnamon**

Begin to heat the oven to 180 ° C. In the meantime, combine the wheat and millet flour in a bowl, the sea salt, yeast and mix well. Clean and peel the pears and cut only the two firmest into thin slices. Set the other two pears aside. Line a pan 20-22 cm in diameter with baking paper and arrange the pear slices on the bottom, overlapping them so that there are no gaps. Then cut the two more ripe pears into small pieces and place them in a mixer bowl. Add the rice milk, the oil, the malt, and the cinnamon and blend well until you obtain a smooth mixture which you will combine with the dry ingredients previously mixed, mixing briefly. Pour everything into the pan on the slices of pear. Bake and cook for 40-45 minutes. Finally, remove the cake from the oven, let it cool for 5-10 minutes before serving it with a vegetable cream sauce sweetened with a few tablespoons of rice malt of about.

6)   Vegan apple pie

Ingredients:
- **3 apples**
- **250 g of type 1 wheat flour**
- **60 g of raisins**
- **60 g of almonds**
- **About 250 ml of apple juice**
- **50 g of corn oil**
- **1 teaspoon of cinnamon**
- **grated lemon peel**
- **1/2 sachet of baking powder**
- **1 pinch of salt**

Soak the raisins. In a bowl, put the dry ingredients: flour, chopped almonds, lemon peel, cinnamon, and salt; stir with care. In another, gather the apple juice, the oil, the raisins, the peeled and chopped apples; mix them well, and mix them with the other container's contents. Mix the mixture carefully, roll it out in a pan; bake at 180 degrees for about 50-60 minutes. Check the cooking with a toothpick: if it comes out dry, turn off the oven. Let the cake rest briefly, unmold it, and let it cool completely on a wire rack before enjoying.

7)   Plum and fig balls

Ingredients:
- **100 g of pitted dried plums**
- **100 g of dried figs**
- **50 g of chopped hazelnuts**
- **cocoa**

Put the plums, figs, and hazelnuts in the mixer. Knead them until you get a homogeneous mixture from which you will obtain slightly larger balls of hazelnuts with the shell. Roll them well in cocoa and immediately arrange them in paper cups. They are ready to be served!

8) Carrot cake

Ingredients:
- **200 g of wholemeal flour**
- **80 g of almonds**
- **80 g of raisins**
- **200 g of carrots**
- **100 g of rice malt**
- **4 tablespoons of sunflower oil**
- **1 orange**
- **3 tablespoons of corn starch**
- **1 teaspoon of yeast**
- **½ teaspoon of natural vanilla**
- **soy milk**
- **1 pinch of salt**

Wash the orange, grate the zest and squeeze the juice. Put the first in a bowl together with the flour, finely ground almonds, starch, yeast, vanilla, and salt. Stir. Mix the oil, malt, and orange juice in a bowl. Gradually add them to the dry ingredients. Complete with grated carrots and rinsed raisins. If the dough is too firm, dilute it with a little soy milk. Line a square mold of about 20 cm on each side with baking paper. Transfer the mixture, level it, and bake at 180 degrees for about 45 minutes. Check the cooking with a toothpick, which must come out dry. Let the cake cool in the pan, turn it out of the mold, and let it cool.

9) Chocolate cake

Ingredients:
- **80 grams of unsweetened cocoa powder**
- **100 grams of coconut flour**
- **300 g 0 flour**
- **100 gr of hazelnuts**
- **150 ml of seed oil**
- **350 grams of rice or soy milk**
- **150 g of cane sugar**
- **a sachet of vanilla yeast for cakes**

In a blender, finely chop the hazelnuts and place them in a large bowl. Add the unsweetened cocoa, coconut flour and flour, sugar, and vanilla yeast. Mix these ingredients vigorously with your hands, mixing them well together. Then add the vegetable milk and mix the mixture with the help of a spoon. Also, add the seed oil: the result must be a soft, not liquid compound. Line a cake pan with parchment paper and spread the cocoa mixture starting from the center towards the outer sides, and spread all the product well in the pan. You can put some chopped hazelnuts or almonds on top of the cake for decoration. Place in a preheated oven at 180 ° for 40 minutes. Remove from the oven and sprinkle the cake while still hot with a coconut flour cascade or, if you prefer, powdered sugar. Few genuine ingredients that, when mixed, give a great result. Excellent for those intolerant to dairy products and to let everyone discover a lively and tasty vegan diet.

10) Quinoa pralines with peach pulp

Ingredients:
- **1 ripe yellow peach**
- **150 g of quinoa**
- **2 tablespoons of brown sugar**
- **7 tablespoons of coconut flour**
- **5 tablespoons of chopped pistachios**

Peel the peach and chop the pulp in the mixer until you get a homogeneous cream that you will put in the fridge. Rinse the quinoa well under running water and cook it in a pot with boiling water for the package's time. When cooked, drain it, put it in a bowl, add the sugar and let it cool completely. Add with the coconut flour and the peach cream until you get a thick and compact mixture that you will work with your hands to make balls with a diameter of about 3-4 centimeters. Roll them in chopped pistachios and put them in the freezer for 20 minutes, then transfer them to the fridge and always serve them cold.

11) Strawberry Tofu Mousse

Ingredients:
- **200 g of natural tofu**
- **250 g of strawberries**
- **3 tablespoons of 100% gluten-free rice or corn malt**
- **chocolate flakes**
- **some mint leaves**
- **1 tablespoon of lemon juice**
- **water as required**

Prepare a mint infusion by leaving the leaves to infuse for at least ten minutes in hot water. Strain it and use that water to boil the tofu together with three tablespoons of malt for a few minutes. After cooking, let the mixture cool in its water to make it flavor well. Drain and blend the tofu with the clean and chopped strawberries and a tablespoon of lemon juice. Use the infusion water to help you combine the tofu and strawberries well and obtain a soft mousse. Pour the cream into the cups and store it in the refrigerator for an hour. Finally, garnish with fresh mint leaves and chocolate flakes.

12) Quinoa truffles with chocolate

Ingredients:
- **100 g of quinoa**
- **200 ml of vegetable milk**
- **200 g of almonds**
- **100 g of whole cane sugar**
- **apple juice**
- **2 teaspoons of flaked agar-agar**
- **2 teaspoons of cocoa powder**
- **1 teaspoon of cinnamon**
- **grated zest of 1 lemon**
- **1 teaspoon of cream of tartar**

Lightly toast the quinoa without using fat and cook it with sugar and vegetable milk (without using the water). Let it swell and cool. Meanwhile, dissolve the agar-agar in a glass of heated apple juice, then add the lemon zest, cinnamon, and cream of tartar. Stir in the chopped almonds, cocoa, and cereal. Let the mixture cool well and then form truffles with the help of a teaspoon. Bake at 180 degrees for 20 minutes.

13) Dark chocolate, almond and matcha mini-cupcakes

Ingredients:
- **200 g of 70% dark chocolate**
- **1 handful of shelled almonds**
- **matcha tea**
- **a few pinches of Himalayan salt**
- **a few pinches of vanilla powder**

Melt the dark chocolate in a double boiler. As soon as it has liquefied, add the chopped or chopped almonds, 2 teaspoons of matcha tea, salt, vanilla, and mix well. Pour the mixture into small molds for chocolates or into muffin molds in which you have inserted cupcake cups. Let it cool to room temperature or in the refrigerator. When the sweets have entirely solidified, decorate them with a sprinkling of matcha tea.

14) Orange cake

Ingredients:
- **300 g of wheat flour 00**
- **150 g of clear raw cane sugar**
- **½ sachet of yeast**
- **the zest and juice of an orange**
- **50 ml of extra virgin olive oil**
- **vanilla sugar to taste**

In a bowl, mix flour, brown sugar, yeast, the grated rind of an orange together with its juice, extra virgin olive oil, and about 100 ml of water. Mix everything with an electric or hand whisk until you get a creamy mixture. Transfer to a pan greased with oil and sprinkled with flour. Bake at 180 degrees for half an hour. When cooked, spread the icing sugar over the cake.

15) Baked stuffed apples

Ingredients:
- **6 apples**
- **1 orange**
- **¾ cup of shelled walnuts**
- **¾ cup of raisins**
- **¼ cup of natural apple juice**
- **1 tablespoon of miso**

Wash and with a knife, starting from the top of the apple, make room for the filling. Heat the oven to 150 °. Rinse the raisins and chop them with the walnuts. Wash the orange and finely grate the zest. Add the orange zest, miso, and a teaspoon to the raisin and nut mixture. Mix well. Stuff the apples with the dough. Arrange the apples in a baking dish. Pierce them with a fork all around so that they do not explode during cooking. Pour the apple and orange juice into the pan and bake in the oven for half an hour. Eat them warm or cold.

www.ingramcontent.com/pod-product-compliance
Lightning Source LLC
Chambersburg PA
CBHW071328130726
47996CB00002B/668